Hamlyn all-colour paperbacks

A. S. Playfair

Modern First Aid

Illustrated by Edward Osmond

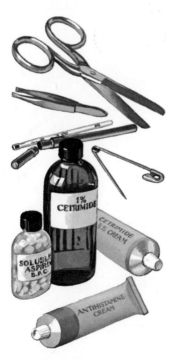

Hamlyn · London

FOREWORD

At any moment anyone may find himself willingly or unwillingly, in the role of first-aider. He may be alone with an injured man. He may be one of a crowd at an accident. At first shy of interfering he will note how most bystanders do just that – stand by. A few rush in to make matters worse. If he is knowledgeable he will drop his diffidence to take over completely.

He may even be the victim himself, and doubly grateful if he understands how to behave.

Each day Great Britain experiences over twelve hundred *serious* accidents. Nearly sixty of them are fatal. Each day four people are killed at work, and twenty on the road. The dear old familiar home is even more dangerous and more people are killed there than in all traffic accidents. Each day twenty-four victims die from home mishaps – an average of one death every hour.

First aid is not a matter for the few. It concerns everyone with a social and personal conscience. That means all of us.

A.S.P.

Published by the Hamlyn Publishing Group Limited
London · New York · Sydney · Toronto
Astronaut House, Feltham, Middlesex, England

Copyright © The Hamlyn Publishing Group Limited 1973

ISBN 0 600 33433 3
Phototypeset by Filmtype Services Limited, Scarborough
Printed in Great Britain by
Sir Joseph Causton and Sons, Limited, Eastleigh

CONTENTS

4	Introduction
5	Shock
22	The Breathing Rate
22	The Pulse Rate
23	Bleeding
38	Burns
44	Wounds
50	Crush Injuries
51	Fractures
66	Sprains and Dislocations
68	Unconsciousness
73	Head Injuries
82	Breathing for Life
87	Resuscitation
88	Artificial Respiration
100	Heart Massage
106	Injuries of Lungs and Chest
111	Electric Shock
116	Poisoning
124	Effects of Temperature Changes
130	Emergency Delivery
135	Minor Nuisances
141	The Car Accident
144	Some Medical Emergencies
152	The Pattern of First Aid
156	Acknowledgements
156	First Aid Courses
156	Books to Study
157	Index

INTRODUCTION

Let this be quite clear: First Aid is FIRST Aid. It is not treatment proper. It is help given to the injured before the doctor or nurse takes over. The term 'First Aid' implies that 'Second Aid' is to follow. We must distinguish between steps to safeguard a patient on the one hand, and the specialized care by medical personnel on the other. To encroach on the latter may interfere with subsequent treatment. It also runs the risk of doing damage, however good the first-aider's intentions and commonsense may be.

There are, of course, plenty of quite minor cases where home care is all that is required; the doctor's time need not be wasted. But this is not first aid. It is domestic therapy.

Calmly and sensibly applied first aid may reduce suffering (as in dressing burns and wounds), prevent an injury from worsening (as in the protection of a fractured spine), begin the road to recovery (as in immobilising a fractured limb). It may save life (as in managing unconsciousness or drowning).

This book has two aims. By means of the index it can be used for quick reference in emergencies. Its main purpose however is to be read for teaching and self-training. Though a little dogmatism is necessary, attempts are made throughout to explain the reasons underlying the actions. With good fortune this may give a subsidiary aim to the work: that of being interesting.

Every student should try to join a group working together. First aid can be learnt by oneself but it is a richer and wiser thing to join a course run by the local branch of one of the three organisations listed on page 156. In collaboration with each other the organisations publish a First Aid Manual on which their training and examination are based. This present book does not pretend to replace the Manual, which is the course text-book. The course consists of eight to ten two-hour sessions at times convenient to most people. The examination which follows is optional. Those who fear facing it can be reassured that the examination is a courteous and kindly affair, of a few minutes only, but sufficient to check that the candidate can justifiably bear the label of qualified first-aider.

If the reader cannot join a course let him teach himself by constant reading and by practising unashamedly on friends and on members of his family. If he takes it seriously, so will they.

No special equipment is needed. It is handy to have a set of bandages and dressings. However mishaps tend to happen when none of this is about. The first aider will learn to be efficient using everyday domestic material.

Pages 152 to 155 are important since they summarise the general principles and management for all cases. These can be read repeatedly with profit to the first-aider and to his future patients.

Badges of St. John, St. Andrew's and Red Cross: centres of first aid teaching

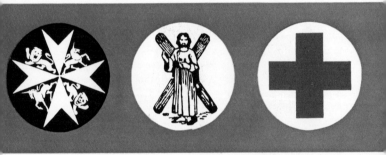

SHOCK

In the world of medicine 'shock' has a very clear definition, quite different from some of the loose meanings of everyday talk.

Two sorts of 'shock' have been described but only one of them really deserves the name.

1. PRIMARY, NERVE OR EMOTIONAL 'SHOCK' is not much more than feeling faint or fainting, a nervous response after injury or a sudden emotional upheaval. It comes on *immediately*, or very soon after the event which provokes it. It is not generally serious and recovery is quick.

2. TRUE SHOCK is quite different – a state of affairs in which the patient's life forces are running downhill. It follows severe injury to the body and *develops gradually*. The consequences can be grave and even fatal. In this book, whenever the word 'shock' appears it is this second type which is meant.

What Causes Shock?

Any severe injury will do this. The most shock-producing calamity is severe bleeding. Extensive burning comes a close second. Severe lacerations, contusions and fractures also can produce shock.

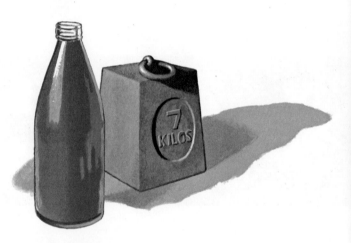

For each stone (7 kilos) of its weight the body contains about one pint ($\frac{1}{2}$ litre) of blood

Bleeding and Shock

For every stone of his weight a human being has one pint of blood. Like all generalisations this is not accurate, but it is a useful guide.

Imagine a fairly petite housewife (she weighs eight stone) who comes to the front door to collect her milk bottles. Four await her. She trips on the bottles, fractures her leg and cuts her wrist. Blood loss is rapid and a pool of red mixes with the white of spilt milk. If she had lost four pints she would be in a very bad way indeed. She would have lost nearly half the total blood in her body. Even if she had lost but two pints she would still be gravely affected.

This example gives some notion of amounts; we are not familiar with a fluid volume when we try to think of it as blood in the body, but have no difficulty in picturing it as milk in bottles.

After bleeding of any severity there is less blood to go round the body. The heart – the pump which keeps the blood moving – automatically tries to compensate by beating faster.

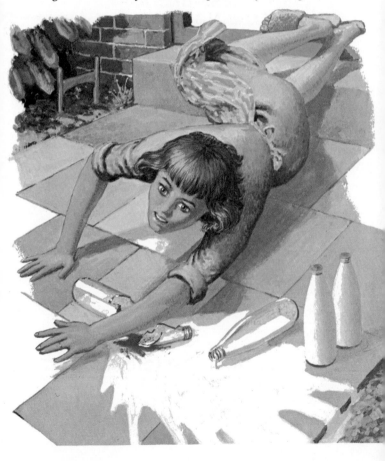

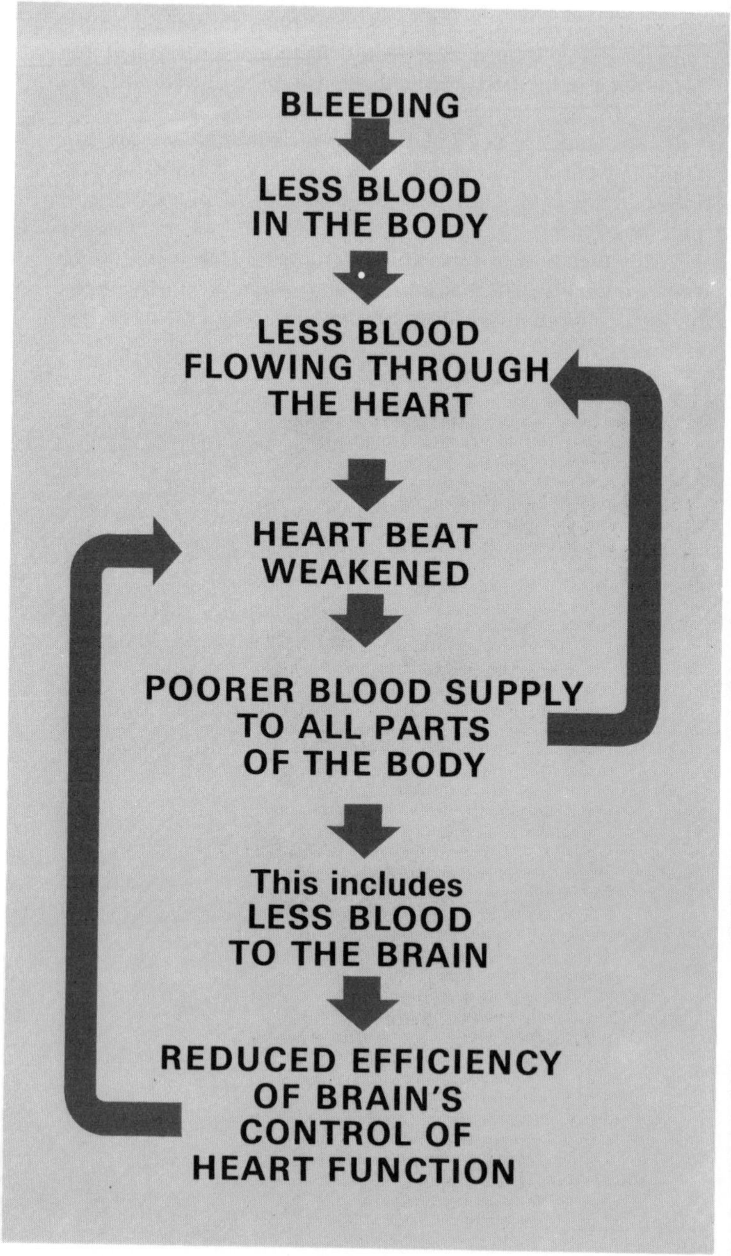

BLEEDING

↓

**LESS BLOOD
IN THE BODY**

↓

**LESS BLOOD
FLOWING THROUGH
THE HEART**

↓

**HEART BEAT
WEAKENED**

↓

**POORER BLOOD SUPPLY
TO ALL PARTS
OF THE BODY**

↓

**This includes
LESS BLOOD
TO THE BRAIN**

↓

**REDUCED EFFICIENCY
OF BRAIN'S
CONTROL OF
HEART FUNCTION**

Though it is doing its best it has to work on insufficient material and it becomes less efficient. As a surgeon put it: 'The motor is spluttering because the tank is running dry'.

The body's reduced amount of blood is now circulating less and less well. Since all tissues depend on a vigorous supply of blood to bring them fresh oxygen and nutrition, the systems and organs of the body, including the brain, will be at lower potency. The brain maintains consciousness. By nerve messages it regulates the working of the heart, lungs and blood vessels. Very sensitive to adverse changes in its blood supply, the brain can quickly lose its competency to control these vital services.

The diagram shows how a vicious circle can set in. This is shock, which can be defined as a state of collapse in which the circulation of the blood is depressed below its capacity to keep the body alive. In severe bleeding therefore *shock is due to loss of blood from the circulation*.

Burns and Shock

We know by experience that a burn may produce a blister. The fluid which fills the blister has come out of the neighbouring blood vessels (page 39). It is in fact a 'watery' part of blood, which oozes through the walls of the vessels to fill up spaces under the damaged skin. This seepage of fluid is one of the characteristics of burnt tissues.

If the skin has been burnt away there remains no roof to form a blister and to contain this fluid which can ooze out in considerable quantity. The wet and messy appearance of the burn testifies to the quantity which is steadily leaking away. All of it has left the blood vessels and is lost to the circulation of the patient. In its own special way, it is a type of 'bleeding'.

Though only the 'watery' part of the blood has been lost it is as important as any other part. The total volume of blood in the body has become correspondingly decreased so setting in train the vicious circle already described.

For burns too we can say: *Shock is due to loss of blood from the circulation*.

The diagram opposite shows how shock develops in a vicious circle of cause and effect

Wounds and Bruising and Shock

Cuts and lacerations are accompanied by bleeding. If the injury is bad, specially if the cut is ragged or deep, we can expect that much more blood has been lost than we can see on the surface. Deep within the tissues blood vessels have been torn to bleed out of sight. The invisible haemorrhage may be considerable.

Some of this blood may show up as bruising. Bruises are collections of blood caught up under the skin. Blue or purple at first, they can with time turn to green or yellow hues. Blood of a wound or bruise is like an iceberg. What we see at the skin may signify much greater amounts lying deeply.

A man may have fallen from quite a height, escaped without a cut or broken bone, and suffered only severe bruising of the chest wall and upper arm. The hollows of one shoulder and arm are puffed out from two pints or more of blood which has escaped from many vessels damaged by the fall.

Similarly one can picture

Bruising is a loss of blood in circulation

the swollen appearance of a badly sprained ankle. We could imitate this shape on a normal ankle by packing it round with jelly. By imagining how much jelly, scooped out of a milk bottle, is needed we get an idea of the volume of blood causing the swelling. To be sure it is still inside the patient's body. But it is taking no part in the circulation.

In the case of wounds and contusions: *Shock is due to loss of blood from the circulation.*

Fractures and Shock

Anyone who has carved a joint will agree that bones do not exist in isolation, but are packed round with meat (muscles) and blood vessels. One cannot break a bone without at the same time tearing some surrounding blood vessels.

A fracture of major bones can be associated with gross damage to arteries or veins, and the diagram shows, in milk bottle terms, the frightening amounts of blood which may be lost in this way. Even if there is no open wound the blood has escaped from the circulation to fill the tissues and to swell the area.

In the case of fractures: *Shock is due to loss of blood from the circulation.*

Fluid volume in swelling

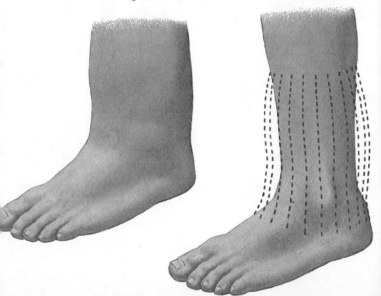

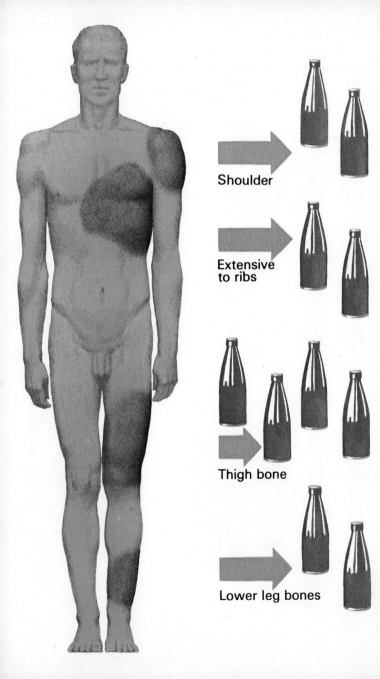

Shoulder

Extensive to ribs

Thigh bone

Lower leg bones

The Shocked Patient

He is pale, or even ash grey.

He is cold to the touch. These two features are partly due to the reduced blood circulation and also to the fact that in shock the blood vessels at the body's surface tend to contract and narrow. They hold within them less blood to colour and warm the skin.

He is sweating. It is an unpleasant cold sweat, like a thin clammy dew.

His breathing is weak, shallow and fast. This is the usual reaction. Sometimes after intense bleeding however the breathing is quite the opposite: deep and gasping, a condition graphically described as 'Air Hunger' (page 32).

The pulse is fast and weak, reflecting the altered beat of the heart. Instead of good firm individual impulses, separate one from another, the pulse has what is known as a 'thready' character. It has little throbs which are fast and run into one another.

He is mentally altered. He may be rather restless in his movements but is likely to be slow in speech, thoughts and reactions. As he worsens he may eventually go into a coma.

He is thirsty. He may request a drink. (But do not give it – see page 21.)

The First Aider's Role

This picture describes shock in its complete state, a desperate situation which should rarely be seen. The first aider cannot cope with it. It is an urgent hospital matter requiring very specialized techniques.

The first aider is not called upon to 'treat for shock'. His job is *to treat to PREVENT* shock.

The injured man with good colour and good pulse must be guarded. He is not beyond danger. He may be just beginning to enter the early stages of shock's vicious circle. It is now that the first aider's actions may save a patient from becoming a sorry statistic.

The diagram opposite shows the possible hidden blood losses which may occur from fractures to certain parts of the body

The Importance of Speed

Picture the development of shock in chart form. Up the vertical part can be marked the 'life forces' ranging from full health (100%) to death (0%). Time is marked along the horizontal part in units which vary according to the circumstances. Whether shock develops in an hour or in many hours after injury depends upon the speed of the blood loss.

The patient was perfectly fit until the point A when he was knocked down and badly hurt with some bleeding. From now on shock starts to develop, represented by the sloping down of the 'life forces' line. At B a first aider has arrived and begins to treat to prevent shock. This is so effective that the fall is halted; the line ceases to descend and straightens out. The patient is in a good condition for medical treatment to his injuries.

If the first aider arrives later or dithers and does not take proper action until C, the downhill run will have gained

The first aider's way of treating may be the deciding factor in that solemn phrase: 'Disposal of the patient'

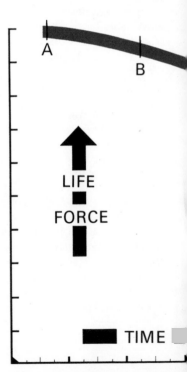

14

momentum and the recovery rate is far slower. The line does not straighten out for a long time and the patient's condition remains very low. Hospital treatment for shock is necessary.

If first aid measures have unfortunately been delayed until D, then it may be too late. The patient's collapse progresses and becomes refractory to even the most careful hospital attention. The outcome may be fatal.

The moral is clear. Do not wait for the signs of shock to appear. For any severe injury immediately undertake the *prevention* of shock. It does not matter if the patient is a powerful-looking person who wishes to over-ride your decisions. Make him obey your instructions.

These could be so good that the patient will remain fit and never even suspect that he owes his recovery to the simple measures of the person who attended him. He may even consider that this person was fussy and officious. He will be mistaken. But he will be alive.

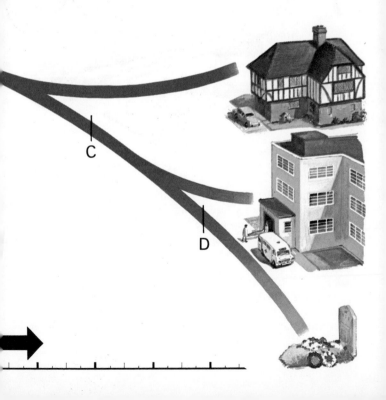

To Prevent Shock

The measures are extremely simple, and may seem to be ordinary everyday common sense actions. So they are. This apparent simplicity might lead the reader to skim the lesson over and not fully learn it. This would be tragic, for on how fully the details are remembered may depend a life.

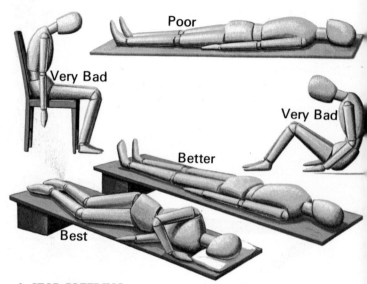

1. STOP BLEEDING

This, the first and foremost move, deserves a special chapter (page 23).

2. ADJUST THE PATIENT TO REST

The body cannot afford to lose any of its energy now. All handling must be very gentle, with special care if there is the possibility of fracture (page 54).

Treat the patient where he is found. If he is in the street attend to him there. If an ambulance is likely to be arriving soon it is best to let him stay where he is.

Of course there are exceptions. The site may be so dangerous that the patient's safety, to say nothing of your own, demands that he be moved: – a house on fire, a gas-filled room or a tottering building. In a road full of moving cars you may be able to instruct bystanders to divert the traffic. Appalling weather could be another reason for shifting the patient.

Lie the patient down even if he plays tough and wants to carry on. Exert your authority with the combination of command, confidence and courtesy which gets results. You will help the patient's blood towards his brain and heart by tilting him with his head low and his legs raised. A flat pillow under the head for comfort is quite in order. The feet need to be no more than about twelve inches high; it does not matter if the slope is a little greater. A few blankets or a greatcoat rolled up can be placed under the legs. A stretcher can be tipped with one end resting on a couple of chairs. The foot of a bed can be propped up on a stool.

Do not keep the patient's face looking skywards. Should he become unconscious his tongue might loll backwards into the throat, blocking the airway to the lungs. Should he be sick (as often happens after injury) some of the vomit might be drawn into the windpipe and cause choking.

Turn him sideways, with his head tilted slightly backwards. This position allows saliva, blood or vomit to flow out

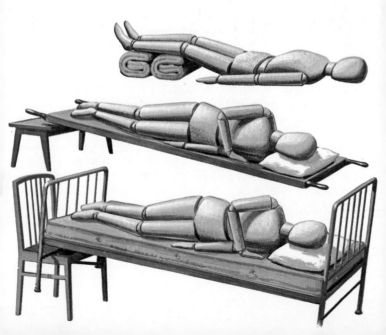

In serious cases the patient's legs can be set up almost vertically, allowing more blood into effective circulation to heart and brain

and prevents the tongue from falling back (see page 68). Should the nature of the injuries compel you to keep the patient on his back, you can at least turn his head sideways. (But beware of doing this if his backbone is fractured; see page 63).

Loosen tight clothing round the neck, waist and chest, so helping the patient to breathe more easily. Neckties, collars, braces, belts and corsets are particularly constrictive when the wearer is lying down. However do not open up clothing more than is necessary.

3. KEEP THE PATIENT WARM

The operative word here is 'keep'. The body's temperature must be maintained, but not raised.

Any pallor which an accident victim shows is partly a protective mechanism. The skin is pale because its blood vessels have contracted and hold very little blood. If the patient is now heated these vessels dilate, fill up with blood, and produce a pink colour. To re-fill those dilated blood vessels takes a great deal of blood, drawn from and denied to the heart and brain areas which need it urgently. Heating your patient with hot water bottles may give him a better complexion, but would increase the speed of shock developing.

All you do is to wrap the patient up in blankets or coats to

KEEP him warm. Tuck these well round and under him; but keep them comfortably loose. If he is lying on a cold surface like the ground or an uncovered stretcher gently get the blankets underneath him as well.

4. RELIEVE DISCOMFORT

Pain and anxiety aggravate developing shock. Their relief is more than just a humane measure; it is a physical necessity.

Cover and dress wounds and burns. Dressings reduce pain and protect against infection (page 45).

Safeguard physical comfort. Do not overdo wrapping up to the point of swaddling the patient tightly. Be guided also by his report on any position which he finds easiest.

Beware of leaving him so that he could roll off a couch and hurt himself further. If circumstances force him to remain there for some time it is wise to have one side of the couch against a wall and bring a suitable piece of furniture against the other side as a barrier.

If he is sweating heavily mop his face gently with a dry cloth.

Safeguard mental rest. Fussing or patting the patient's hand or brow will only increase his apprehension. Bystanders and relatives are liable to cause confusion by disorganised acts

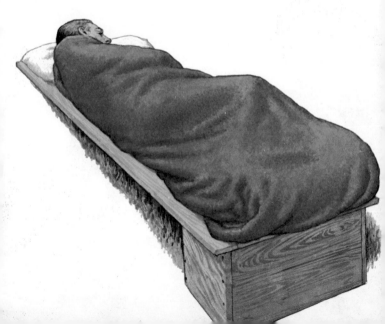

which reflect their own panic. Dispose of or dismiss agitated watchers as best you can. Request them to perform some task which gets them away from the scene. Bringing water (which you may not really need) to the boil or carrying messages of minor importance will give them time to calm down.

It is extremely unpleasant for the accident victim to find himself lying helpless at the feet of strangers staring down with morbid curiosity. The old cry of 'Give him air' is absurd as it is unlikely that a crowd could prevent air reaching him. The real value of clearing away bystanders is psychological. On the other hand the constant presence of a first-aider who is acting calmly and confidently is a great factor of reassurance. Keep talking to him quietly and sensibly. Well-meant but vague platitudes such as reiterating 'There, there, don't worry' cause disquiet. The anxious man who is told not to worry can but conclude that there is something sinister to worry about.

He may ask questions about his condition. Answer directly, but use your skill to do this without giving away how badly he may be hurt. Keep up the note that you have the situation in hand and that further help is on its way.

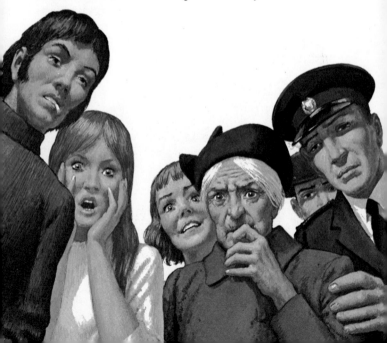

A man who has been crushed asks tremulously: 'Will I lose my leg?' The first-aider secretly fears that this may indeed be so. He replies in such terms as: 'I am sorry your leg hurts so much. But I have dressed the wound and you are not bleeding now. The leg is splinted so that it can come to no more harm. An ambulance is coming and you will soon have the doctor's help'. The question has been tackled, but with deviation giving only positive and comforting statements.

The patient may be unduly anxious about points which to you seem of lesser importance: 'Where is the parcel I was carrying?'; 'Where is the girl who was with me in the car?'; 'Will you inform my wife?' (or 'Please do not tell my wife'). Do not dismiss these, but satisfy him as best you can.

Discretion is an essential quality. Do not discuss the case with others in the patient's hearing. With the unconscious the sense of hearing was the last to go and will be the first to return. Always act as if the apparently unconscious man can overhear. On the other hand do not whisper to others in his presence; he will at once assume the worst.

Nothing by Mouth

Never try to give anything by mouth to an unconscious man. He cannot swallow properly and fluid given may choke him.

Even when the patient is conscious the rule holds that one should not give anything by mouth. This may seem unnecessarily cruel to a man who is likely to be thirsty. Yet fluid can remain some hours in the toneless stomach of the injured man, only to be vomited up later; if at the time he is unconscious, or under an anaesthetic at hospital, the vomit might choke him.

If the patient asks for a drink it is kinder to tell him that this must await a doctor's permission. In the meantime slight relief could be given by letting him suck a clean handkerchief moistened with water and wrung out. He will refresh his dry mouth without getting any significant volume of fluid into his stomach.

Alcohol must be condemned as a false stimulant. In any quantity it has the effect of widely dilating the blood vessels of the skin. In this respect it acts as dangerously as would the wrong use of hot water bottles by drawing blood away from the brain and heart.

PREVENTION OF SHOCK–SUMMARY

1 STOP BLEEDING

2 ADJUST TO REST

Minimise movement   Gentle handling

Patient lying down: head low, feet raised

Tight clothing loosened

3 KEEP PATIENT WARM

Covers above and below him

No extra heat needed

4 RELIEVE DISCOMFORT

Dress wounds and burns

Safeguard physical comfort

Safeguard mental comfort

FORBIDDEN: Anything by mouth

THE BREATHING RATE

The rate of respiration at rest is about 12 to 16 a minute. But excitement and exertion can bring it up much higher. It is easy to count, watching the rise and fall of a bit of clothing on the chest. Practise discreetly on companions in halls or trains; it is even simpler to do on a patient who is lying still.

THE PULSE RATE

The pulse is an impulse in an artery corresponding to each beat of the heart. It is felt where a convenient artery lies between bone and skin. Immediately in front of the notch of the ear is a handy place when the patient is fully covered up. The more usual site is a couple of finger breadths above the crease of the wrist, on the palm and the thumb sides. Feel with two or three fingertips over the artery. Do not use the less sensitive thumb. Do not press hard – just enough to feel the throbs. Slightly bending the patient's hand down at the wrist relaxes ligaments near the artery, and makes the pulse more easily felt.

Practise regularly; get to know the feel of the normal pulse. Learn to do this on people who are lying down without moving or disturbing their arms.

The normal adult pulse is about 70 a minute, but there can be quite big variations in health, with a range from 60 to 80. As shock develops the rate may eventually reach about 150. When attending to a badly injured man it is wise to keep a timed and written record of the pulse every few minutes.

In young children the pulse rate is faster. The *average* rate for the new-born baby is 130, for the two-year old it is 100 and for the seven-year old it is 90.

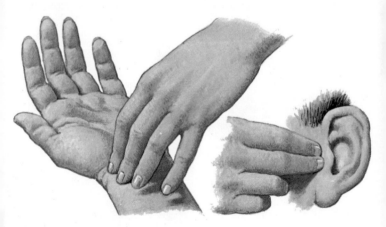

BLEEDING

The body contains about ten pints of blood, or roughly a pint per stone of body weight. The average adult who loses rapidly two pints or more is in difficulties which threaten his life.

When bleeding occurs microscopic fibres form within the fluid of the blood at the site of injury. Eventually they form an entangling meshwork, the clot, which closes the breach in the blood vessel. By reducing the blood flow at the wound we help the clot to form. We prevent its breakaway by keeping the treated part at rest.

Mild bleeding, the nick from shaving, the grazed knee, the cut finger, will eventually stop by itself if left alone. Dressing it firmly as a simple wound (page 44) will generally stop it at once.

Stopping Severe Bleeding

When bleeding is so profuse that the patient is in danger act promptly: RAISE THE BLEEDING PART, where this is practicable, to reduce the force of the flow. If the hand is bleeding bring it above the head. (This must not be done when you suspect a fracture; a broken bone must not be moved.) APPLY PRESSURE TO THE WOUND. Boldly and quickly use your fingers and thumb to close the wound and to hold its edges firmly together. Do not be afraid of grasping hard. Pressing

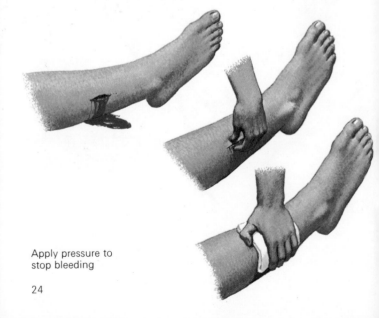

Apply pressure to
stop bleeding

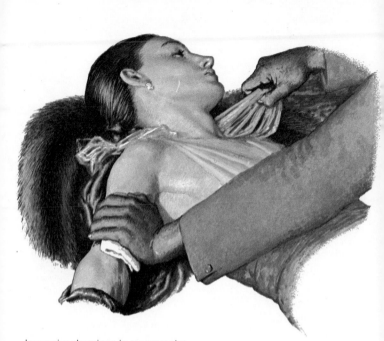

Improvise dressings in emergencies

down with the fingers may be enough. Do not wash your hands first; the risk of infection is less important than that of haemorrhage. MAINTAIN PRESSURE WITHOUT RELAXING FOR TEN MINUTES to allow the clot to form. Try to keep the pressure up while you manage the next steps. GET THE PATIENT LYING DOWN as soon as you can. PRESS A BIG DRESSING OVER THE WOUND and hold it there while you put a thick pad of material over it. Where the wound is open and deep pack the dressing pad well into it. It will be useless if it merely bridges over the wound. Secure the whole with a firm bandage.

If you are alone with the patient improvise with what is about you. With your free hand fish about your person and pockets (or the patient's) to obtain handkerchief, scarf or necktie. If you do have to let go to rush for dressings, then you must hope that your ten minutes' pressure has allowed formation of

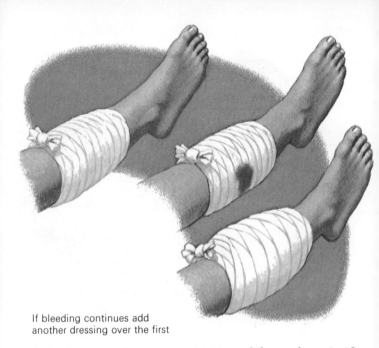

If bleeding continues add
another dressing over the first

a clot firm enough to stay in position while you leave it. If others are about hold onto the wound until they bring you napkins, towels or proper dressings and bandages.

Pressure should be over the wound but not encircling the whole part. Forbidden is the tight tourniquet which constricts round a limb and can be very dangerous, depriving the whole of the limb of its blood supply. Only at the bleeding stump of an amputation (fortunately very rare) is a tourniquet permissible.

NOW PUT THE PART AT REST, KEEPING IT ELEVATED IF POSSIBLE. A leg or arm can be supported up on a stool or on pillows. The patient remains lying down and you attend to his other needs to prevent or reduce shock.

WATCH FOR FURTHER BLEEDING. If the bandage shows a growing stain of blood do not take it off and so disturb what partial clotting may have taken place. Apply more padding and another firm bandage over the stain. If blood oozes into this second cover apply a third.

Special Types of Bleeding
Ear Bleeding

A cut outer shell or the lobe of the ear may bleed fairly freely. Sit the patient up ('elevate the bleeding part'). Grasp the cut firmly through a layer of thin clean material for ten minutes. Let a co-operative patient do the grasping. When the bleeding has stopped put on a firm pad and bandage.

Bleeding from inside the ear canal is a different matter. The loss is likely to be slight but the conditions which cause it must be treated with respect. A scratch or boil of the canal may bleed. The ear drum at the far end of the canal will bleed if it ruptures. Infection may do this. So may a sudden increase of air pressure from the blast of close gunfire, a box on the ear or diving into water.

A fractured base of skull sometimes shows up with bleeding from the ear, for only a thin layer of bone separates the ear canal from the brain above it. IN ANY CASE WHERE BLEEDING FROM THE EAR FOLLOWS A BLOW ON THE HEAD ALWAYS THINK OF THE POSSIBILITY OF A FRACTURED BASE OF SKULL (page 74). A loss of watery fluid (from the clear liquid which surrounds the brain tissue) suggests the same thing.

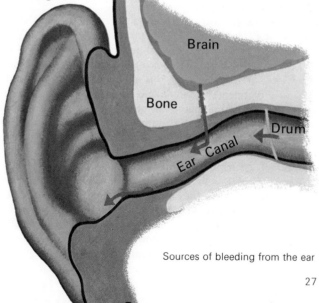

Sources of bleeding from the ear

What not to do is more important than what to do. Never put in drops; they could carry the infection to inner parts. Never plug the ear hole with wool; this blood must be allowed to escape. If it accumulates it might encourage infection since it forms a splendid source of nutrition for any microbes present.

The whole outside ear is covered with a clean dry dressing which is bandaged in position. If bleeding is copious (this is rare) lie the patient with the ear downwards to encourage the blood to flow out, but remember to avoid pressure on any possibly fractured part.

Nose Bleeding

Diseases which cause nose bleeds include catarrh and raised blood pressure. Injuries as causes range from the child's nose scratching to a broken nose or even a fractured base of skull. The top of the inside of the nose has only a very fine bony partition between it and the brain. As with ear bleeding REMEMBER THE POSSIBILITY OF A FRACTURED BASE OF SKULL WHENEVER NOSE BLEEDING OR WATERY FLUID LOSS FOLLOWS A BLOW TO THE HEAD.

Proper first aid will almost always stop nose bleeding though it is worth while later to get a doctor's advice when it comes without obvious reason.

Where there is no likelihood of a fractured skull sit the patient up ('elevate the bleeding part'). Bend his head slightly forward to prevent blood trickling down the back of the throat. Put a towel round his neck and have a basin handy to catch any further dripping. This organised care improves the patient's morale. The whole lower nose is pinched firmly between finger and thumb for at least ten minutes. Let the patient do this himself. He can make himself comfortable by resting his elbow on the table. If bleeding recurs repeat the process.

Common errors are pinching the bony upper bridge of the nose instead of the soft part at the nostrils, and not keeping an unrelaxing grasp for the proper time. The patient must not swallow or blow his nose; these actions disturb clot formation.

If the patient is unconscious lie him down with his head to one side to allow the blood to flow out and to prevent it trickling from the back of his mouth into his windpipe.

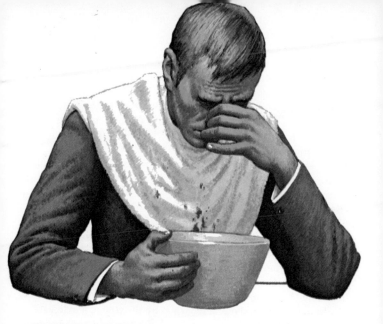

Bleeding from the Tongue

One can bite one's tongue deeply. A smoker may fall and cut his tongue on a broken pipe stem.

Sit the patient up and use a towel and basin (as for nose bleeding). Grip the tongue through a clean handkerchief between the thumb and finger. Press firmly without relaxing for ten minutes. Let the patient take the grip himself. If the patient is unconscious lie him down, as for nose bleeding.

Bleeding from a Tooth Socket

This may happen a few hours after a tooth extraction. The mouth should not be washed out during the bleeding. This mistake would displace clots which are trying to form. Sit the patient up and use the towel and basin as for nose bleeding. Place a generously thick cotton wool or gauze plug on the socket area (but not into the socket which would harm it).

Now the patient bites hard on the plug and keeps this up for ten minutes. He will find it less tiring if he rests his jaw in a cupped hand, with the elbow on a table.

Bleeding from Lungs

Blood may be coughed up in small streaks, sometimes mixed with phlegm. The strain of repeated coughing can produce a spot of blood. Heavier bleeding may come from diseases or injuries in the chest. In this case the blood will be frothy and bright red, characteristics given it by the air in the lungs.

If only a slight amount of blood is coughed up this is a problem for the doctor who MUST be visited or called in according to the patient's condition.

Where bleeding is heavy the patient must be taken to hospital without delay. The important features of lung injuries and haemorrhage are described on page 106.

Bleeding from the Stomach

The most likely cause is a poison or a disease such as an ulcer which has eroded a blood vessel in the stomach wall.

Bleeding may be slow and insidious, with blood accumulating gradually in the stomach before it causes sufficient upset to make the patient vomit. While pooling there (minutes or perhaps even hours) it is acted upon by the stomach's digestive

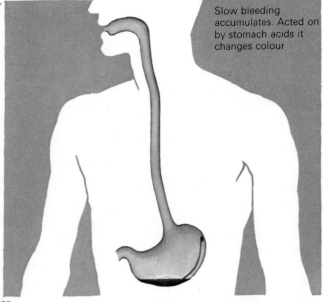

Slow bleeding accumulates. Acted on by stomach acids it changes colour

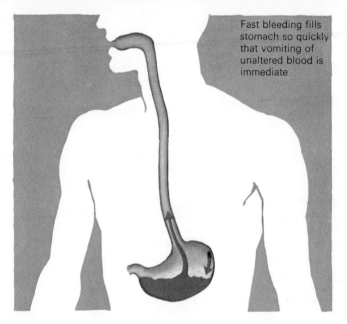

Fast bleeding fills stomach so quickly that vomiting of unaltered blood is immediate

juices which turn its colour from red to brown or nearly black. When it is vomited it may not look at all like blood but exactly like coffee grounds. BLACK VOMIT INDICATES BLEEDING IN THE STOMACH AND NEEDS IMMEDIATE MEDICAL ATTENTION.

If a large stomach vessel is affected blood may fill the stomach so fast that the patient is sick almost at once. There has been no time for reactions with digestive juices and the blood comes out true red. A common error is to think that all haemorrhage from the stomach looks like dark coffee grounds. *The colour depends on how long it has been lying in the stomach before it has been vomited.*

Whether slow or fast this bleeding is not necessarily painful, and may cause but a mildly queasy feeling. Meantime the patient may be losing enough to become deeply shocked.

Treatment is simple and urgent. The patient must be lying on his side with the head low, and kept at absolute rest. Full anti-shock measures are taken (page 16), and medical help is needed at once.

Internal (Concealed) Bleeding

This is bleeding with blood accumulating within the space of the abdomen or chest and not showing up outside. It may be caused by disease or by crushes and blows – a car crash, a fall from a height, or blast. A small puncture wound may overlie dangerous damage.

Severe blood loss can take place without its being obvious except by its effect of rapidly developing shock and you must be on the alert to recognise it.

The patient may or may not be in pain. A rigidly-firm belly is suggestive of severe internal trouble; the muscles have hardened as an automatic protective measure. Bruising of the abdominal wall is also a danger sign.

Be on your guard as soon as a patient becomes abnormally restless. His pallor may become startling or turn to a dusky hue. The clammy perspiration of shock will be marked, and so will the coldness of the skin, especially at the hands and the tip of the nose. Soon the weakness and speed of the pulse makes it difficult to be felt. Respiration is not the shallow sort of more slowly developing shock. It is fast, laboured and sighing; this has the expressive name of 'Air Hunger'. The patient is very thirsty. Voices of those around seem to him far away; he may have buzzing noises in his ears. He may complain that everything seems dark and misty.

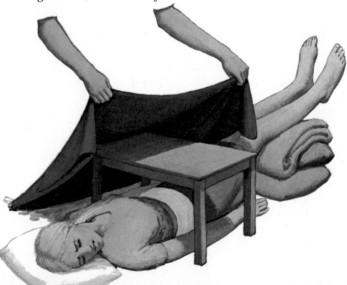

Not all these features may be present; but any set of them form a serious picture of collapse. Treatment is as for preventing shock (page 16) with a great sense of urgency. The patient needs a transfusion and must be sent to hospital at once; every moment counts. He must be kept at rest lying down; with his legs raised and with his head low and turned to one side. Covering is important, but should be arranged to avoid heavy weights on the abdomen. Nothing must be given by mouth.

Bleeding from Varicose Veins

In the leg veins valves which allow one way flow towards the heart break up the distending pressure on the vein walls of this long blood column. Muscle movements help the blood flow, but in the immobile standing leg the blood tends to bulge out the veins so that the valves can no longer close up. Successively lower sections of the vein are involved. A badly-distended vein lying just under the skin is vulnerable and may rupture from a blow or strain. Bleeding is profuse and the patient may panic.

Treatment is easy. Press your hand on the bleeding

point and keep it there. Lie the patient down and elevate his leg, resting the heel on a chair edge. Remove tight bands like garters. Replace the pressure of your hand with a clean pad such as a well-folded handerchief and bandage this on firmly, making sure it does not slip.

Heavy Bleeding from Forearm, Wrist and Hand

A few years ago the first-aid world rejected methods of trying to control bleeding by compressing pressure points. These were specific sites where an artery lay closely under the skin and passed over bone. Firm pressure here could occlude the vessel by squashing it against the underlying bone. It was held that fumbling for these anatomical sites, ill-remembered and tricky to find, could be an ineffectual and a dangerous waste of effort compared to the method taught today.

However there are two pressure points in the arm worth learning (and, indeed, one has returned to official acceptance). Of all parts of the body the hand and forearm are most susceptible to bad injury. We handle machines and cutting tools all too carelessly. In danger we place our arms protectively ahead of us. The use of these pressure points is for the dangerous and fast haemorrhage which could result, and not for simple bleeding easily controlled by other means.

The large artery supplying forearm and hand runs down

the upper arm along a line corresponding to the inner seam of a sleeve. It lies along a hollow between two fat muscle bands, rather like a river flowing in a valley between two hill ranges. It overlies the bone against which it can be pressed.

You can demonstrate its site by having someone standing below a lamp and trying to bend his elbow while you try to hold his arm straight; as the muscles tense up the 'valley' shows up as a shadow between them.

To control heavy dangerous bleeding in the elbow and fore-arm or hand:

1. Straighten and elevate the patient's arm.
2. Cup your hand under the upper arm, your fingers curling round its inner side so that the finger tips fall naturally into the 'valley'.
3. Press the finger tips down against the bone.

The second pressure point is a little lower where the artery runs across the thin and bony front of the elbow. If the elbow is bent right up the artery is compressed between the bones forming the joint. In addition it is kinked and blocks itself, like a thin hose pipe which is folded back. This works better

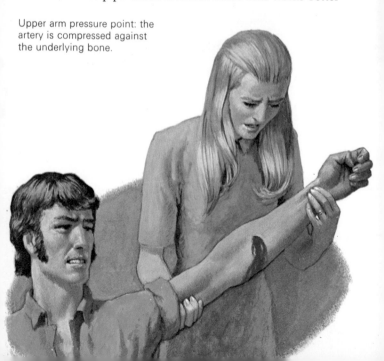

Upper arm pressure point: the artery is compressed against the underlying bone.

(Left) Flexing the elbow against a firm pad controls bleeding of forearm or hand. (Below) A pad is clenched in a cut palm to control bleeding

if there is time to stuff a pad, like a bunched up handkerchief, in the elbow fold.

If you feel your own pulse at the wrist and then bend the elbow up very firmly you will note how the pulse disappears because the artery has become blocked.

There are two reservations about both these pressure points. This method is unsuitable for fractured arms, since broken bones must not be moved or handled hard. Also the artery should not be blocked longer than ten or fifteen minutes since this would have the same detrimental effect as the forbidden tourniquet. But those minutes will allow clotting and the correct application of a firm dressing and bandage at the bleeding site.

Bleeding from the Palm

A wound here may bleed freely. Direct pressure should control it well and the patient can exercise this himself with the minimum of trouble. A pad rolled into sausage thickness is placed over the dressing (a roll of two-inch bandage is ideal). The patient closes his fist hard over it. The whole hand is then firmly bandaged in this position and kept elevated.

A Note on the Functions of Blood

Why do we have blood? Of what use is this fluid?

It does for the body what road and railway traffic does for the country, the city, the road or the house in which we live. The analogy is a fair one. Factories, shops and larders depend on the vehicles which carry goods to and from them. Blood is a communication and transport system for nutrition and chemicals. Every organ, every tissue, every cell depends on blood for life and protection. *Blood vessels* are the 'motorways' through which this 'transport traffic', the *blood itself*, passes. The functions of the blood and its components are as many and varied as are those of railway carriages, lorries, delivery boys on bicycles, postmen or policemen on foot and refuse carts to be seen on our roads.

However the nation would weather a transport strike for quite a while before collapsing for lack of materials and communication. Not so the body; it cannot afford to be deprived of blood for any but the briefest of moments.

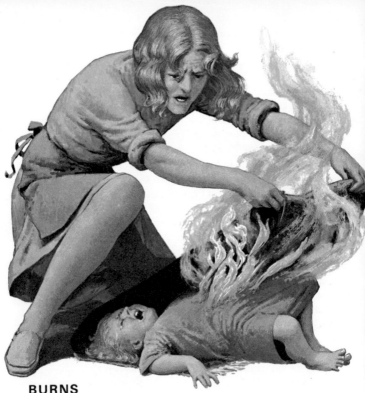

BURNS

Clothes on Fire

The patient may be running about terrified, so fanning the flames which can flare up towards his face. All too often this is a child, victim of an unguarded fire.

GET THE PATIENT ON THE GROUND AT ONCE. If he is panicking this may have to be done by tripping him up. This is no time for courtesies. If you can manage it get the patient lying with the burning part uppermost to prevent the ascending flames licking round the body. SMOTHER THE FIRE by wrapping round firmly and closely a thick cloth or blanket. Do not delay to fetch this – grab any rug or cushion immediately available or use a hastily whipped-off coat or skirt. Protect the patient's face by bringing this smothering object down to fan the fire away from the head and towards the feet. Manipulate it also as a shield between yourself and the flaming patient.

Do *not* roll the patient round and round on the floor. This would expose all sides of the body to upward rising flames. Rolling to extinguish flames is the last resort of the burning man who is alone with no-one to help him.

Clothes Merely Smouldering

Smothering these under thick covering would press the heat into the patient's skin. Where possible tear off the smouldering bits, holding them at non-burning parts. Stamp them out at once.

The Damage Caused by Burns

A simple scorch, showing a surface redness, heats deeply beneath the skin damaging the blood vessels. These react by dilating and also by becoming permeable, letting the colourless fluid part of the blood ooze out through their walls to distend the surrounding area. Lifting up the thinned deadened skin at the centre of the burn, the fluid forms a bulging blister. The volume of the blister is but a small index of all the fluid lost from the blood vessels and lying soggily in the depths.

A more severe burn destroys the whole surface of the skin leaving an open wound. There is no longer any 'roof' to contain liquid within a blister. This wound is wet from the unhindered flow of fluid and much may pour and continue to pour out of the burn.

The area of a burn is more significant than its depth. When a large surface is damaged many more blood vessels are in-

Healthy skin   Scorch becoming a blister   Open burn

Various burns

volved, with a great volume of fluid flowing out and therefore a high risk of shock.

First Aid to Burns

IMMERSE THE BURNT PART IN COLD WATER IMMEDIATELY. Cooling will lessen the pain. It will reduce the heat still held within the tissues. The cold reverses the burn reaction by making the blood vessels narrow down again and decreasing the loss of fluid through their walls.

Put the part under a running cold tap while you fill a sink or bucket. Then plunge the burn into the water. If this is impossible, as when dealing with chest or abdominal burns, drench the area with cold water and maintain this with wet cloths. Renew the cloths as they lose their coldness. It is no use pouring on a little water and leaving it at that. Thorough soaking is needed. Immersion must be continued for at least ten minutes and as long as there is pain.

(Opposite) From a photograph: when a child scalded her arm someone immediately plunged it into cold water. This however reached elbow level only. Forty years later the contrast of healthy and scarred skin teaches its lesson

Do not go to the extreme of using iced or cold water, for this degree of cold is quite unnecessary and can be really painful. Do not further hurt the burned site by spraying the water on as a powerful jet.

In severe cases keep the patient lying down and use ANTI-SHOCK MEASURES.

REMOVE ANYTHING CONSTRICTIVE. Bracelets, rings or garters may cause a lot of trouble if swelling develops.

DRESS THE BURN AS FOR WOUNDS with clean dry materials, once the area has been well cooled and not before. Infection is a potent cause of later scarring. Do not risk infection by piercing blisters, but leave them alone. (But see also p. 140.) If any burnt bits of material are adhering to the wound leave them there. Removing them would hurt, and they can be considered as sterilised by the heat; loose cloth around them should be cut away.

KEEP THE BURNT PART ELEVATED if this is practicable for it helps to reduce the swelling. A hand, for instance, can be set up in a sling or kept high on pillows.

In severe cases it is wiser to send the patient to hospital urgently than to delay by

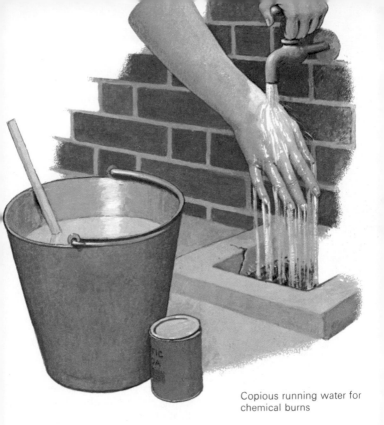

Copious running water for
chemical burns

waiting for a doctor to come. While waiting for the ambulance you may give fluids provided the patient is conscious. Do this cautiously: a small cup of tepid water every ten minutes, sipped slowly, will be right. Anything more carries the risk of inducing vomiting.

Scalds and Hot Fat
Clothes saturated in steam, boiling water or hot fat will continue to burn the skin unless they are taken off rapidly.

Chemical Burns
Strong acids and alkalis can burn the skin as badly as can flames. Rapidly remove any clothes wet with these (but take

care of your hands!). DILUTE AND WASH AWAY THE CHEMICAL by a copious continuing stream of running water until there is no likelihood of any remaining. On no account try experiments such as neutralising acid with alkali or vice versa. This would waste time and increase the insult to injured tissues by using them as a receptacle for uncontrolled chemical reactions.

Scalds of the Mouth and Throat
These are dangerous for the loose tissues here can swell with speed, blocking the airway and causing choking. REPEATED SIPPING OF COLD WATER OR SUCKING ICE may be tried. A wet cold compress round the neck offers slight further help. But aim principally to get the cooling at the back and inside of the mouth.

Friction Burns
Harsh rubbing from a machine or from sliding down a rope can cause the same effect as ordinary burns and needs the same treatment.

Electrical Burns
The burn may show as a small dark area at the point of contact. Under the skin however the electricity will have fanned out deeply into a wedge of burnt tissue. Since electricity closes up blood vessels in the area this small outer mark may overlie a wide zone of dying flesh which deserves medical attention.

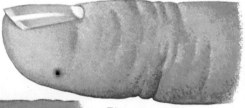

Electrical burn

WOUNDS

Dressing a wound properly achieves four things: controlling bleeding; protecting against infection from the entry of germs through the breach of the skin; reducing pain at the exposed nerve endings; allowing best conditions for ultimate healing.

A simple cut will mend with minimal scarring if the edges are kept clean and in apposition. Grazes, being quite superficial, should also heal well. Lacerated and ragged wounds are much more prone to become infected and form unpleasant scars. A puncture wound, as from a nail or sharp prong, may show as but a small depressed point on the surface. Beneath it lies deeply the menace of important structures damaged and of infection driven in. Its innocent outer aspect is misleading and a doctor's opinion should be sought.

First Aid to Wounds

CONTROL ANY SEVERE BLEEDING AT ONCE.

WASH YOUR HANDS THOROUGHLY – a point which is often overlooked. While you are doing this and preparing for

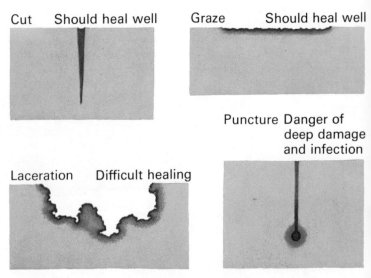

Cut Should heal well

Graze Should heal well

Puncture Danger of deep damage and infection

Laceration Difficult healing

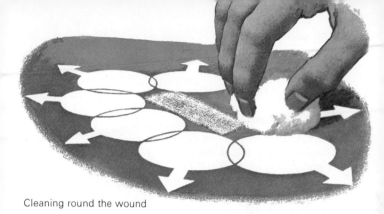

Cleaning round the wound

the next steps keep a temporary cover on the wound. The untouched inside surface of a clean towel or handkerchief will do.

CLEAN THE SKIN AROUND THE WOUND with small swabs of gauze or wool moistened in soap and water (or in the Cetrimide solution referred to on page 48). Carry the dirt away from the area by making overlapping strokes moving outwards from near the wound edge, but never touching the open wound. Use a fresh swab for each stroke.

If the wound is quite small as on a fingertip there is no objection to holding it under a gently-flowing tap. In most places tap water can be considered as germ-free.

COVER THE WOUND WITH A DRESSING. Ideally this should be gauze from a freshly-opened packet. It must be generously big to extend well beyond the wound on to the clean skin. Most beginners make their dressings too small so that a slight shift would expose the wound.

If gauze is not to hand you may use the smooth surface of lint. Never use the irritant woolly side, and never cotton wool. But every household has a supply of emergency dressings in its cupboards: handkerchiefs, smooth towels, pillow cases and napkins. Washed and ironed each has been stored clean with its inner folds the next best thing to being sterile. Hold it up carefully by the edges and let it fall open; still handling only the edges refold it so that what had been the inside unexposed layer now becomes the outside. Do not let it touch anything before you lay it on the wound.

Specially-prepared adhesive dressings are excellent for

small wounds. Peel their backings off carefully so that your fingers do not touch the central gauze strip.

COVER THE DRESSING WITH A THICK PAD of cotton wool or any suitable material such as clean handkerchiefs. The pad acts as a buffer against blows and also soaks up any discharge which may come from the wound. It must be thick enough to absorb this fluid without letting it reach its upper surface. Otherwise germs may track from the outside through the moisture into the wound.

BANDAGE THE WHOLE FIRMLY, but not too tightly. A common mistake however is loose bandaging which will slip or unravel. In emergency work it matters little if the bandage looks irregular and ungainly. As long as it keeps the dressing secure and comfortable it is doing its task.

Ordinary woven bandages are very suitable but crepe bandages, with their elastic properties, are better. Apply them slightly on the stretch to hold the dressing with gentle pressure. If you have no bandages improvise with stockings, small towels, large handkerchiefs or even scarves and neckties.

Dressings recommended for the first aid set are described on page 154.

Special Wound Problems
Dirt Lying on the Wound
This can be gently brushed off with swabs immediately before cleaning round the wound.

Embedded Objects
Do not try to remove them; this is a task for the doctor or nurse. Place the dressing gauze loosely over the wound. Over this build up a trough of cotton wool padding to surround and project well above the embedded object. Further padding and bandaging now goes on without danger of pressing it in. To prevent its moving and causing further harm put the injured part at rest.

Bullet and Shrapnel Wounds
A bullet or a flying fragment which enters with force may remain within the body. Beware of assuming that this is so. It may have passed through (often with an erratic course) to tear

The wound with an embedded object has to be specially protected before bandaging

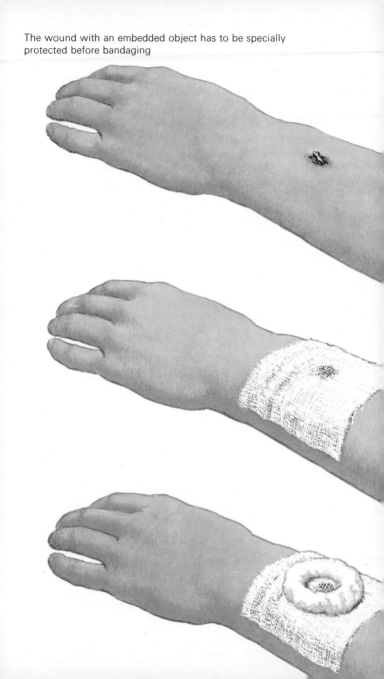

an exit hole considerably bigger than the entrance wound. Very gently explore the patient for this possibility. You may find a large second wound needing attention.

Do not use Antiseptics

Many antiseptics are detrimental to the open tissues. Their use must be left to the doctors and nurses who will take over subsequent treatment or 'second aid'.

However if a wound is a slight domestic affair, not to be brought to experts for further attention, then it is reasonable to use a carefully-chosen antiseptic. One such is 1% *Cetrimide Solution*. This is obtainable from chemists and should be kept in a small sealed bottle. It must not be used after seven days of opening the container. The same solution is very effective, instead of soap and water, for cleaning skin round the wound. $\frac{1}{2}$% Cetrimide Cream is also available, and is useful for spreading on dressings to prevent them from sticking.

The Risk of Tetanus (Lockjaw)

This infection lurks everywhere and particularly where a wound is contaminated with soil or comes from an animal's bite or scratch. It is also likely to arise in puncture wounds: the jab from a garden fork and even the deep prick of a rose thorn carry the danger. Do not hesitate to get medical advice if there is the slightest doubt.

Wounds of the Eye

Do not put in any drops for these might irritate. Bandage a dressing and a large soft pad over the whole eye.

If the eye is badly hurt or has an object embedded in it you must avoid pressure on it and you must keep it from moving. Since the two eyes move as one the only way to do this is to put the good eye at rest as well by blindfolding the patient. Explain to him why you do this otherwise he may fear that both are injured.

Abdominal Wounds

Such wounds can be very serious and they may be accompanied by internal bleeding (page 32); they need urgent hospital help.

While awaiting the ambulance try to relax the patient's

abdominal muscles. Stretched and tense they might pull the wound open. Put him on his back with his hips and knees well bent up over cushions or rolled blankets or coats. Loosen the trouser top and any tight vest. Turn the head to one side so that any vomit may escape easily from the mouth.

Should any of the abdominal contents project from the wound leave it alone apart from covering it with a large dressing. Do not bandage tightly. In all this expose the abdomen as little as possible.

If the abdomen has been pierced by some object like a knife, a branch or an arrow leave it in position. Its removal could be very damaging, and is a hospital job.

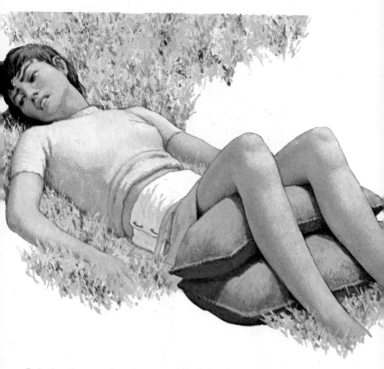

Relaxing the muscles of a wounded abdominal wall

CRUSH INJURIES

A limb severely crushed under a heavy weight for a long time (two hours or more) may look deceptively normal on release. Within a few hours it may swell considerably from fluid oozing through the walls of its blood vessels. This leads to shock.

Reduce the ooze by elevating the limb and by firm – not tight – bandaging with a 3″ crêpe or elastic bandage, applied slightly stretched, each turn well overlapping the previous one. (Do not bandage if a fracture is suspected.) Cover the limb, but very lightly, for if warmed the blood vessels would dilate all the more.

Should there be an unavoidable delay of some hours before the patient reaches hospital you may give the patient some fluid to drink. Do this as you would for burns (page 42).

Chest Injuries

These are dealt with on page 106.

Coordination of muscle action

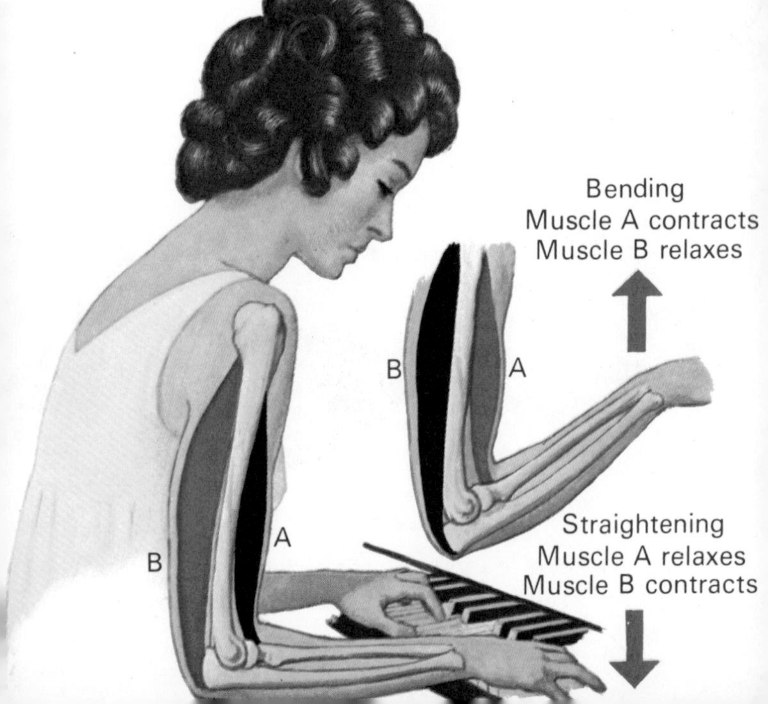

Bending
Muscle A contracts
Muscle B relaxes

Straightening
Muscle A relaxes
Muscle B contracts

FRACTURES

Bones are the girders which support our body. They move upon one another through the contractions of muscles attached to them. The surfaces of bones are not at all smooth, but knobbed and ridged where the muscles are fixed; these irregularities are testimony to muscular pull.

Movements of the elbow show well how mobility is controlled. One set of muscles runs from the shoulder and upper arm bone above to the front of a forearm bone just below the elbow; its contraction pulls up the forearm and bends the elbow. A similar set of muscles at the back of the limb could straighten the elbow again. When the bending muscles contract the straightening ones automatically relax, and vice versa, otherwise there would be a tug-of-war between the two sets and movement would be blocked. In other words bones and joints are constantly subjected to muscle pulls adjusting to each other. These forces balance nicely provided the bone is intact. If the bone is broken its separate parts may be pulled out of line and the limb deformed.

The occurrence of a fracture can be classified as:

1. DIRECT, when the bone breaks at the point where it receives the blow: a heel broken from a heavy landing after a jump;

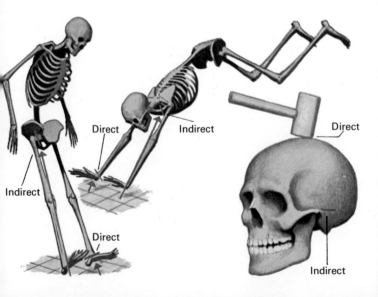

a wrist fractured from a fall on the outstretched arm; a crack where the skull is hit.

2. INDIRECT, when the fracture occurs some distance from the site of the blow. In the landing from a high jump the force may travel up the leg and snap the thigh bone at its top where it is angled to enter the hip joint. The force from falling on the wrist may be conducted through the shoulder to jolt and snap the collar bone. A hit on the dome of the head can crack the lower, hidden, base of the skull. This 'indirectness' must not lead you to overlook fractures some distance from the obvious injury.

3. 'SPONTANEOUS' is the name given to a fracture which has happened with no apparent cause from the slightest of blows. This is rare and involves bones already weakened by some disease.

4. MUSCULAR. It rarely happens that sudden muscle exertion by an athletic person can be so violent as to break a bone.

Another very important classification concerns the relationships of the broken bone to its neighbouring parts.

1. CLOSED. All fractures risk damaging the tissues packed around them. But as long as the skin is unbroken the area remains protected from outside dirt and infection.

2. OPEN. On the other hand the fracture may be in contact with a break of the skin and is therefore at risk of infection. There may be a deep wound or a bullet track leading to the

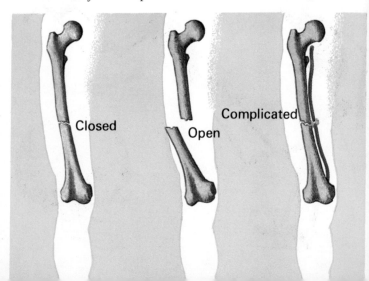

Closed   Open   Complicated

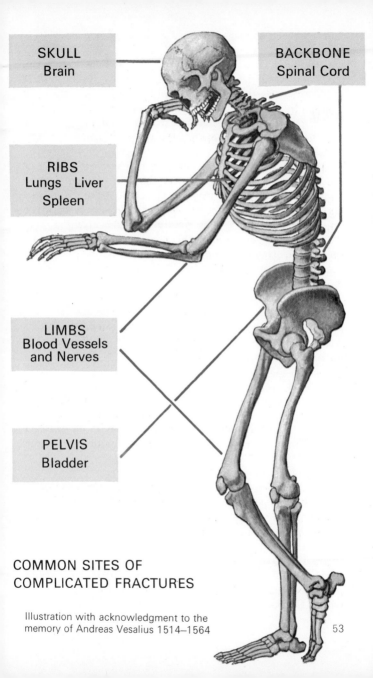

SKULL
Brain

BACKBONE
Spinal Cord

RIBS
Lungs   Liver
Spleen

LIMBS
Blood Vessels
and Nerves

PELVIS
Bladder

COMMON SITES OF
COMPLICATED FRACTURES

Illustration with acknowledgment to the
memory of Andreas Vesalius 1514–1564

53

fracture. Or the jagged end of a displaced bone may have pierced the skin.

3. COMPLICATED. We recognise that no bone can break without some damage to the tissues against it and to their blood vessels (page 11). When this involves an important adjoining structure the fracture is complicated. Remember this possibility of secondary troubles and that far more serious harm could happen to the soft parts than to the bone itself.

SUSPECT A FRACTURE when there has been a blow or crush followed by pain. However the pain is often surprisingly slight. The patient may not be able to move the injured part properly. It may be swollen and deformed, or in an unnatural position. Feeling gently over the area you find that it is tender and (unless this is masked by swelling) that there is an irregular 'knobbliness' which is not present on the opposite side of the body. But you must never try to move it.

If you have any doubts your line of action is clear. Play safe and treat as if there were a fracture. The accidents departments of hospitals are full of carefully-tended patients whose doctors are unashamedly uncertain of the diagnosis until X-Rays make it clear.

First Aid

Our aim is to prevent clumsy movement and handling. The shift of jagged bone ends would certainly cause pain. It could also turn a closed fracture into an open one, or an ordinary fracture into a complicated one, sometimes with very serious results.

1. Control any severe bleeding immediately.
2. Tell the patient not to move. Treat him where he is.
3. Cover any open wound with a light dressing.
4. Immobilise the injured part.
5. Take anti-shock measures.

Immobilisation

Understanding the following principles is better than trying to master, and then forgetting, detailed instructions for each part of the body.

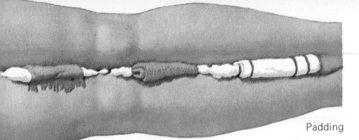

Padding

Immobilise not only the fractured area, but also well beyond the joints either side of the damaged bone.

In most cases the injured part is secured by bandages against a suitable part of the patient's body; fractured arm to the chest wall; fractured leg to the good leg.

Move the good leg to line up against the injured one, rather than the other way round.

If circumstances force you to move an arm or leg into position for securing it, do this slowly and in a planned way. Tell the patient to keep as relaxed as he can. Cradle and support the whole injured limb in both your arms and hands and move it gently and smoothly as one piece.

To prevent uncomfortable pressure and chafing and to increase the stability of the splinting, the hollows of the immobilised limb should be filled up with padding between it and whatever it is secured against. Cotton wool, socks, stockings, handkerchiefs, or small towels will serve. Even tussocks of grass can be used.

A fractured limb is bound in its immobilised position with broad bandages, strapping, stockings or towels which are carefully passed round without disturbance. The bandaging is firm, but not tight and, of course, avoids the fractured site itself. It is tied off with reef knots or with bows which must be on the side of the uninjured part.

In a limb the pressure of a broken bone against a blood vessel could impede circulation. So could compression from severe swelling. But tight bandages and over-thick, hard padding can do this too. The extremity of the limb becomes white, dusky-blue, cold or numb. You can test by pressing on a nail to make it white. On release its pinkness should return quickly. If it remains discoloured check your pads and bandages.

Do not waste time and material on too much immobilisation. If your patient's journey to hospital will be easy and quick simplify procedures. Just be satisfied that he travels without movement of the fracture. A co-operative patient may lie safely with the weight of a rolled-up coat or blanket set alongside the broken limb, immobilising it against the appropriate part of the body. Empty the pockets of anything which could press uncomfortably against the immobilised patient.

Collar Bone

The weight of the arm pulls down the outer end of the broken bone. The shoulder may look flattened and the patient may be supporting the elbow on the injured side to relieve this pull.

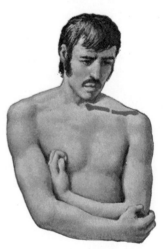

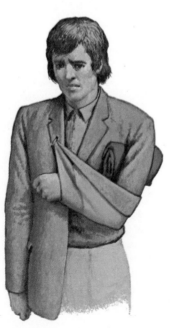

A soft pad is placed in the armpit, and the forearm gently brought over the chest.

Immobilise with the elbow well supported and the hand towards the opposite shoulder, perhaps rather higher than shown in the illustration.

56

Upper Arm, Forearm, Wrist and Hand

Place a large soft pad in the armpit. The forearm and arm are carefully brought across the chest, the hand reaching the opposite armpit.

However if the elbow is painful when you attempt to bend it, keep it straight; the patient must travel on a stretcher in this case.

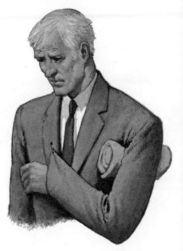

Padding between the limb and the body. Broad bandages round (1) the upper arm and the body, (2) just below the elbow and the body, (3) the wrist and thigh

Ribs

It is quite common for a rib to crack. The patient finds breathing movements painful and therefore takes shallow breaths only. The chest wall muscles support the broken bone wall and no special measure is needed, unless the patient feels more comfortable with his arm in a sling.

See also page 106 concerning more serious chest injuries.

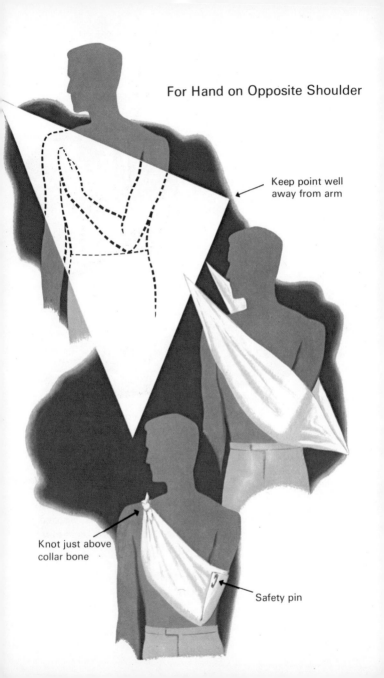

For Hand on Opposite Shoulder

Keep point well away from arm

Knot just above collar bone

Safety pin

Slings

As the examples have shown slings can be improvised by using the patient's clothes. The prepared sling is a triangular piece of cloth, its long side about five feet. But scarves, towels or belts can be used instead.

Take care to keep the patient's arm well supported while applying the sling.

A slight upwards slope to the supported arm not only is more comfortable but also tends to reduce swelling. Slings are likely to stretch so that eventually the arm may sag downwards with it. Watch for this and correct it if necessary.

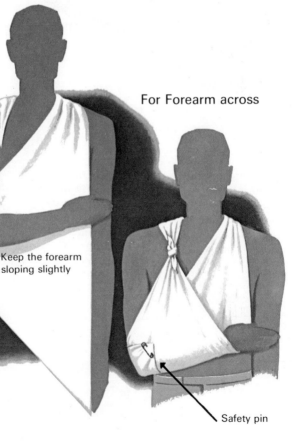

For Forearm across

Keep the forearm
sloping slightly

Safety pin

Thigh and Leg
Bring the good leg alongside the injured one.

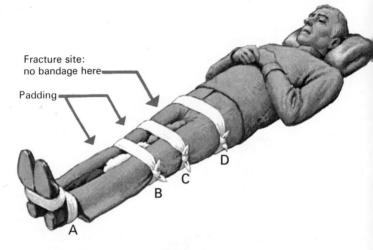

Fracture site:
no bandage here

Padding

(A) First tie the feet and ankles together (by figure-of-eight bandage). (B) Then bandage the knees together. (C) Tie one bandage just below the fracture. (D) Tie one round the thighs

A fracture of the upper end of the thigh bone sometimes (not always) shows a characteristic deformity. Unbalanced muscle pull on the bone below the fracture site may roll the whole leg outwards, the foot being turned sideways on the ground as the patient is lying down.

In the elderly who have deficient bone strength, this is a common fracture after a relatively slight fall or stumble. The

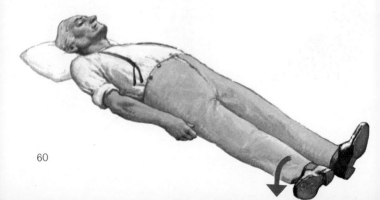

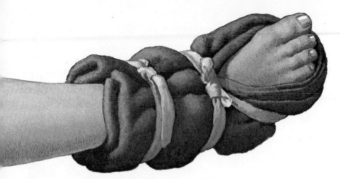
Cushioning the fractured foot

pain may not be severe and if the abnormal position of the leg is present it is a guide to diagnosis.

As the bone is broken high up there is no room for a bandage above the fracture site.

Foot

Gently remove the shoe and stocking or sock. Swelling will be reduced if you keep the foot elevated on pillows or a rolled-up blanket.

A useful protection for the unshod foot and ankle is to tie a pillow or thickly folded blanket round it.

Jaw

Bandaging here is difficult and more often than not ineffectual. The attached muscles will usually tighten in spasm and give enough immobilisation.

If bleeding is heavy there is a risk of blood running back to cause choking. Therefore keep the patient bending forward over a basin. If he is unconscious the recovery position (page 71) is essential. The tongue is attached to the front of the jaw; if this bit has been loosened by fractures on either side, the tongue may slip back with it into the back of the mouth and obstruct breathing. Keep the jaw forward with your fingers hooked over the teeth.

Skull
See page 73.

Pelvis (Hip Bones)

Some hip bone fractures are difficult to distinguish from those of the upper end of the thigh bone. This does not matter; the treatment is as for the latter. More serious fractures can crush and disrupt the bony ring which forms the pelvis. Suspect this when there is much bruising and swelling round the hip and groin, and when pain prevents the patient's moving not only the leg but also the trunk.

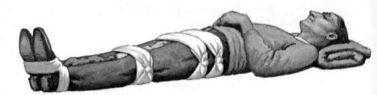

1. Two broad bandages, overlapping each other, go round the pelvis. 2. Padding goes between the legs. 3. A figure-of-eight bandage secures ankles and feet together. 4. The knees are bandaged together.

Let the patient lie on his back and put his legs in the most comfortable position. Bending thighs and knees, for instance, relaxes muscle pull on the broken bones; support the bent knees with pillows or rolled blankets. Keep him thus until the ambulance arrives.

If there is a long wait or difficult travel ahead then immobilisation is needed.

Severe pelvis fracture may injure the bladder or the passage leading from it, making the patient feel he must pass urine. Should he do so urine could leak under the skin at the groin causing further damage. In all pelvis fractures tell the patient he must try not to pass urine until he is in hospital care.

Spine

Each of the chain of bones which form the backbone is made up of a thick plate with projections around it for muscle attachment. In the centre a large hole forms a bony ring through which passes the spinal cord of nerves governing movement and sensation throughout the body.

Injury of the spinal cord, a serious fracture complication, is rare since most fractures of the spine concern only the outer projections of the bone. However if any of the ring itself is broken there is risk of loose bone slipping into the spinal cord and injuring it. Extensive paralysis or loss of feeling could result. It is very important to realise that though the fracture could do this damage at once the patient's rescuer might himself be the cause. The bone might be broken but its loose bits not displaced . . . yet. Mishandling the patient could allow them to shift into the spinal cord. Consider every injury to the back as a possible fractured spine, and every fractured spine as a potential ravager of the cord.

You must prevent the spine from bending forward. Keeping it straight protects against untoward movement of the broken bits. On no account let any would-be helpers pick him up and carry him 'folded'.

Immediately tell the patient to lie quite still until expert help is available, even if this means a long wait. In the meantime cover him with blankets or coats. Test for paralysis by asking him to move fingers and toes, and for loss of feeling by touching his hands and ankles.

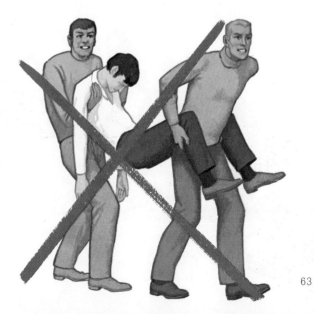

Only if medical or trained ambulance help will not be available – but not by yourself. At least three (and preferably six) others are needed. All your actions must be understood and planned in advance.

First the patient's legs are gently straightened, the two being moved together, since this disturbs the spinal column least. Now put pads between the ankles, knees and thighs. At these three sites tie the legs together with broad bandages (use a figure of eight bandaging at the ankles and feet).

One first aider grasps the head (cupping his hands over the ears) and another the feet. These two *must* remain at their task during all the following moves, maintaining a firm pull which stretches the patient and prevents any twist to the neck and back.

The length of a strong blanket, half rolled-up, is placed alongside the patient. The first-aiders gently turn the patient on his side. The roll is brought close to him. He is turned back over it onto his other side. The blanket is now unrolled flat and the patient turned back to lie on it. (Empty his coat and trouser pockets before these manoeuvres).

A stretcher is brought alongside the patient and pads put on

THE FRACTURED SPINE 1:
The men at each end maintain their pull on the patient until he is safely on the stretcher.

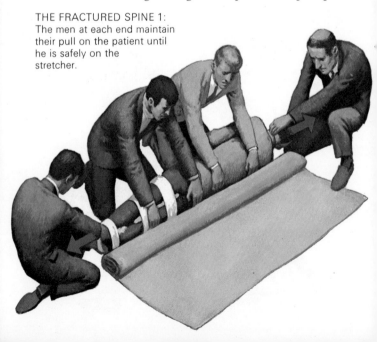

it at positions corresponding to the hollows of the neck, back and ankles. It is now shifted to the patient's feet. The first-aiders roll both edges of the blanket up to the sides of the patient. Grasping these rolls as if they were handles they lift up the blanket, keeping it taut by pulling, and bring him gently over and then down onto the stretcher. All must work in unison to make this a smooth move. It helps if there is one first-aider available to slide the stretcher under the lifted blanket.

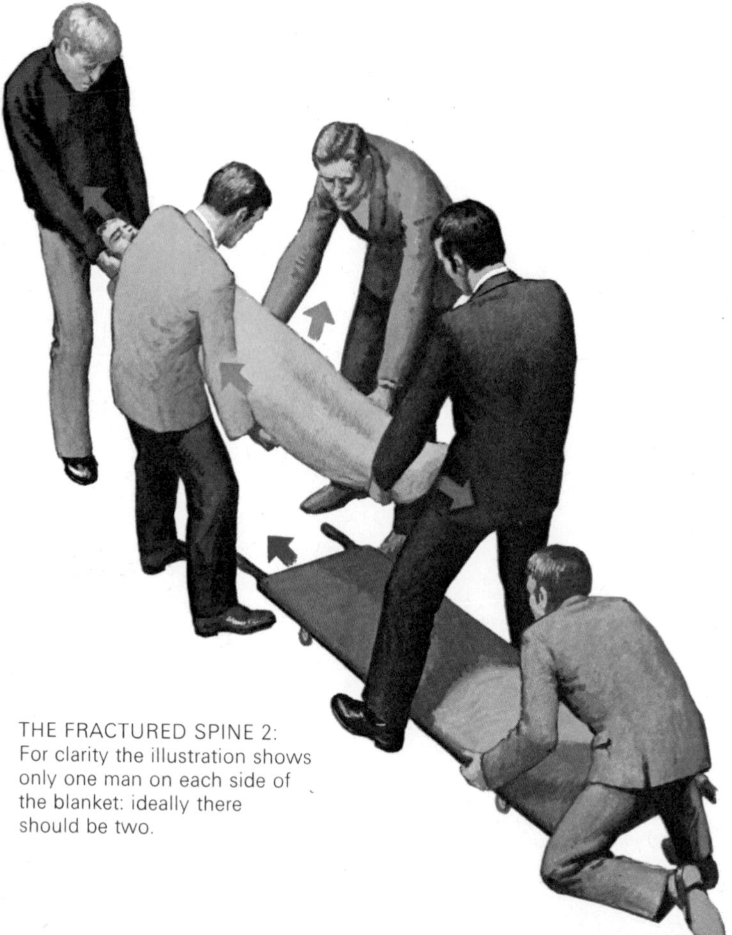

THE FRACTURED SPINE 2:
For clarity the illustration shows only one man on each side of the blanket: ideally there should be two.

SPRAINS AND DISLOCATIONS

Joints are places where bone links with bone, so that movement can take place. The joints are buttressed by muscles and by strong ligaments which keep the bones in position. A SPRAIN is a stretching and tearing of ligaments from a wrench of the joint. A DISLOCATION is a wrench which has gone a step further. Not only has it torn the ligaments but also it has displaced one bone from its normal position against the other.

The diagrams teach that there is no clear dividing line between causes of sprained, fractured or dislocated joints. Their pain, swelling and deformity are very similar. The first-aider

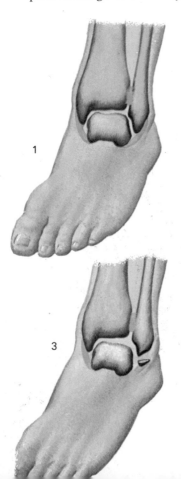

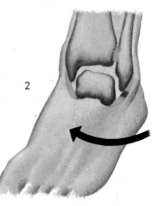

1. *Ankle joint.* Two bones of the leg encase a rear bone of the foot. Ligaments (green) between the bones maintain their stability.

2. *A sprain.* The foot has been wrenched to one side, dragging and tearing the ligament of the opposite side.

3. A sprain which was so forceful that the ligament detached and pulled away with it a tiny fragment of bone. Technically this is a fracture, but the break of the bone is trivial and should mend without difficulty.

cannot make the diagnosis (nor, in many cases, can the doctor without X Rays).

TREAT THESE CONDITIONS AS FRACTURES. Never try to correct a suspected dislocation. Put the joint at rest and keep it supported in the position most comfortable to the patient. This generally means a sling for an upper limb and a stretcher for lower limb injury.

Some important nerves and blood vessels run close to joints and could be compressed by a dislocated bone. Numbness or tingling of the hand or foot could result. The sooner such cases reach hospital the better.

Very mild sprains however may be helped by comfortably firm bandaging over thick layers of cotton wool: use a crepe or elastic bandage over the wool. If you are on the scene just after the injury, try first to minimise the swelling: wrap on for half an hour a cold compress. This is a folded cloth soaked in cold water, then wrung so that it is only moist. As it warms up on the patient it should be renewed.

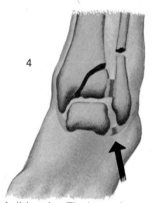

4. *A fractured ankle* from force applied upwards (landing heavily on the heel). Two leg bones are broken near the joint. This cannot help involving some of the attached ligaments, which will be torn. A fractured joint is almost certainly also a sprained joint.

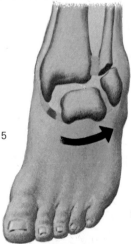

5. *A dislocation*. The lowest bone has been knocked sideways out of its position at the joint. The forced displacement inevitably tore the ligaments holding it. In this particular case it has also knocked and broken one of the bones alongside it. A dislocation is always a sprain as well, and it may sometimes also cause a fracture.

UNCONSCIOUSNESS

To find out why the patient has lost consciousness is the doctor's responsibility. The first-aider's task is to keep the patient alive for the doctor.

It is extremely easy for an unconscious man to suffocate unless he is properly looked after. If he is on his back blood, vomit or saliva may move from the mouth into the windpipe. Dentures or loosened teeth could block the back of the throat. But the commonest obstruction is the patient's own tongue. The thick and fleshy tongue is attached to the front of the jaw bone. We are all familiar with its forward motion, but less aware how far it can move backwards. During unconsciousness the muscles, including those of the tongue, become flabby. If the patient is on his back the limp tongue falls against the opening of the windpipe. Air cannot get past. (This does not happen in ordinary sleep where the tongue keeps its healthy tone).

Three things will overcome these dangers:–
1. *Keeping the head down and to one side* allows fluid to flow out.
2. *Tilting the head back as far as it will go*, with the nostrils pointing directly up, opens the airway at the throat.
3. *Pushing the jaw well forward*, so that the lower teeth project beyond the upper teeth, pulls the tongue clear of the windpipe. This can be done by pulling or by pushing the jaw bone:

Do not underestimate the importance of these simple actions. Always fear obstructed breathing in the unconscious. If the patient is making gurgling or snoring ('stertorous') noises urgent action is needed.

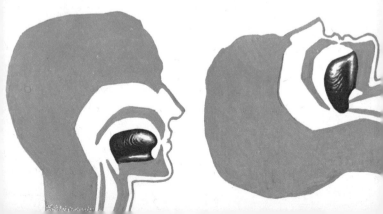

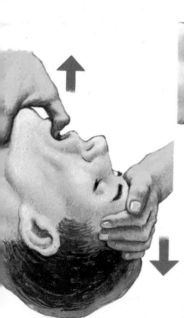

Two ways of maintaining the clear airway. A thumb hooked round the lower teeth pulls the jaw, or fingers behind the angle of the jaw push it forwards. Meantime the head is bent well back so that the nostrils point straight upwards.

Coping with the Unconscious

1. Is the patient breathing? If not give artificial respiration at once (page 88).
2. Protect against choking. He may be trying to breathe but unable to because of airway obstruction. Always check the mouth: with fingers or a handkerchief clear the mouth of anything in it, blood, vomit, dentures, loose teeth.
3. If the patient is breathing properly and not vomiting you should, before moving him, quickly check that there is no deformity indicating a fracture. Feel gently but firmly along spine, limbs and pelvis. If you suspect major fractures (e.g. spine) which forbid your moving him stay by his head guarding the airway, and leave out the next step.
4. Turn the patient into the *recovery position*. Lie him down on one side.

The above are not separate slow items. The good first aider makes them one combined operation.

To get the unconscious patient from his back onto his side first empty his pockets and remove his wrist watch. Then from a kneeling position alongside him:

1. cross his further foot over his nearer ankle;
2. line his arms alongside the body but tuck his nearer hand and forearm well into his side;
3. kneel further back to leave a space into which to turn him.
4. your one hand cradles the nearer side of his face to protect it as it meets the floor, your other grasps his further hip and rolls him over towards you. (If he is too heavy for you to manage this as a single move start by using both your hands to pull him half over onto your knees.)

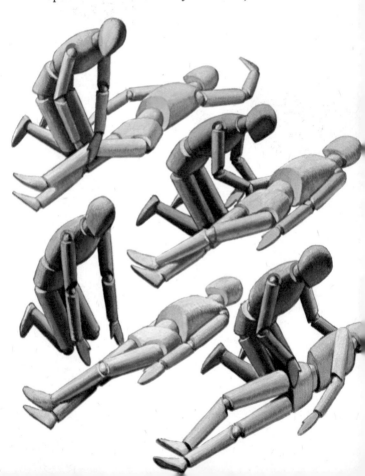

THE RECOVERY POSITION
Lying on one side.
Head bent back; face bent down.
Upper arm bent at right angle at shoulder
and elbow; upper hand near the face.
Upper leg bent at right angle at hip and knee.
Lower arm and leg stretched out behind.

The recovery position keeps the patient supported, with his airway open and allows any fluid in the mouth to flow out. You never know when he will suddenly vomit, and he may do this dangerously and silently.

If the patient is on the ground put a thin clean cloth or handkerchief under his head. But never use a pillow which would raise the head.

Remember that the recovery position applies not only to the sudden accident, but also to the sick man who becomes unconscious in bed.

5. Dress any wounds which you may find.
6. Apply the usual anti-shock measures. Loosen tight clothing, keep the patient warm by covers, tip a stretcher or bed with head end down. While you wait for the ambulance or the doctor watch the patient closely. No one should try to give an unconscious man anything to drink; he might choke.

It is by no means stupid to try to speak to the unconscious casualty. He may be more aware then you know and grateful to receive encouraging words. He may even surprise you by some form of response.

Bleeding and Breathing
If both bleeding and obstructed breathing present a simultaneous problem quickly clear the airway first. This is an easy and rapidly successful move. Immediately after, attend to the bleeding, which may need more care and time. (See also page 95.)

Why Unconscious?
Once you have ensured his safety then, and only then, may you try to assess the cause of his condition. Did he fall? Has he bleeding from ears or nose? (page 74). Is his colour blue (air lack or blood loss) or abnormally red (page 100); look at nose tip or ears for colour. Are there marks of corrosives on the face (page 118) or poison containers nearby? Are the pupils unequal (page 77) or both very small or both very dilated from drug overdose? Does his breath smell of petrol (page 118) or of alcohol? Beware of thinking that alcohol is the cause of unconsciousness. It may be only the cause of the clumsiness which caused a fall and a serious injury. Does he have on him

a card or wrist band indicating that he suffers from diabetes or epilepsy or that he is on special drugs?

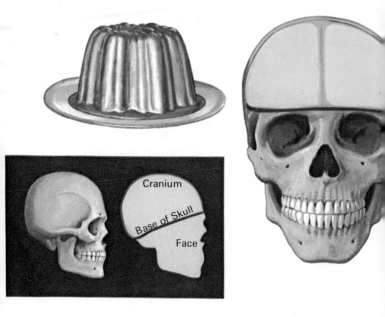

Cranium
Base of Skull
Face

HEAD INJURIES

The skull can be divided into the facial part in front and below and the cranium, or 'brain pan' above. The brain is set within the dome of the cranium and sits on the bony base of the skull. However when we speak of a fractured skull we generally refer to that part which houses the brain.

The very soft substance of the brain is held in its bony box like a jelly set between a hard mould at the top and a firm plate at the bottom. Both brain and jelly fill their containers fully. There is no room for anything extra inside without squashing or disrupting this soft stuff. A serious blow on the mould may shake up or tear the jelly inside. It might break the top of the mould or its force could be transmitted down to break the plate below. The cranium, the brain and the base of the skull can react to injury in exactly the same way.

Concussion

A blow to the head which shakes up the jelly-soft brain may cause a 'knock out'. *Immediately* after being hit the patient becomes unconscious, perhaps for a brief moment, perhaps for minutes, perhaps for hours. When he comes to he feels dazed, but if the concussion was only a mild one then he should recover fully. Sometimes his mind may remain a blank for events leading up to the accident.

On regaining consciousness many insist that they feel fine and wish to carry on. This must not be allowed. For there may be more damage than the first effects suggest.

Fractured Skull

When a skull is fractured it may be either at the point on which it was hit or far away at the base of the skull. It is most important to remember that some parts of the base of the skull are extremely thin and vulnerable, especially round the eyes,

This blow can break the bone beneath it

or at some point at the base of the skull

A fractured base of skull **may** give bleeding from the nose or ear, or **may** give bruising around the eye nose and ears. If your patient shows bleeding or bruising at these points after a blow on the head, always recognise the possibility of a fractured base of skull. Blood is not the only warning. A sticky watery flow may be the escape of fluid which normally lies within the membranes clothing the brain.

The skin overlying a fracture generally becomes puffy quite quickly, so that any irregularity of the bone cannot be easily felt. A bone fragment may be pushed in and press on the brain. The fracture may have damaged blood vessels, which then bleed within the skull.

If the blow has made a wound of the scalp or forehead the danger of an open fracture, with its threat of brain infection, is very real. Even a small cut carries this risk, and what appears trivial may mask a track leading to extensive damage beneath.

All these features compel you to show great caution when coping with head injuries.

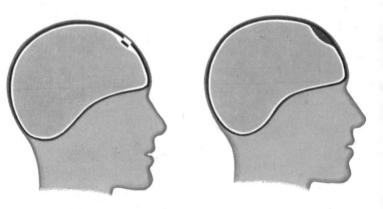

From depressed bone   COMPRESSION   From bleeding

Brain Compression

Two things may compress the soft brain after a head injury. *A depressed fragment of bone* from a fractured skull can weigh against the brain beneath it. *Blood from a torn vessel* within the skull would have the same effect. Quite a minor blow to the head can cause bleeding. If bleeding continues the pressure worsens as the blood slowly takes up space. Tightly fitted within its rigid bony box, the brain tissue can only submit to being increasingly squashed.

Death could be the final stage, the result of compression

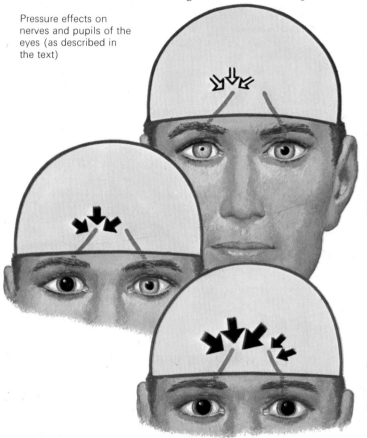

Pressure effects on nerves and pupils of the eyes (as described in the text)

inhibiting those parts of the brain which control such life factors as the heart beat, breathing, temperature regulation and blood pressure.

To some extent the strain upon the brain tissues of the patient can be judged by the behaviour of his mind, of his eyes and of his pulse rate.

The mind. At first the patient may be conscious, though complaining of headache. If compression increases he gradually becomes confused, then will not talk or answer properly, and so becomes more and more comatose until he is completely unconscious.

The eyes. Sometimes (not always) the victim's eyes show signs characteristic of increasing compression. Within the skull are nerves which control the size of the pupils (the dark centres of the eyes). Abnormal pressure on the nerve to one eye can at first stimulate it, making the pupil of that eye contract to quite a small black circle. If pressure builds up further the nerve eventually is overtasked and weakens. The pupil becomes paralysed, dilating into a large black circle. It then no longer gives the normal reaction of contracting when a light is shone into it. In either case the two eyes show pupils of different sizes.

Severe advanced compression may finally affect the nerves of both sides, making both pupils widely dilated.

Equal pupils after a head injury do not prove anything. Unequal pupils, or those which do not contract to light, are very suggestive of brain compression, especially if the size of one or both has been changing on repeated comparisons.

Beware of using undue force trying to prise open eyelids of a face which is severely battered and swollen.

The pulse rate. Increasing compression may inhibit that part of the brain which governs the heart beat. The pulse then slows progressively as the patient moves into unconsciousness. The strength of the pulse however generally remains normal.

Shock is rare. The amount of bleeding within the skull which produces compression signs is quite small. If the patient appears to be developing shock (page 13) suspect that you have missed finding some other injury. For very often accidents to the head are accompanied by damage to other parts of the body.

Concussion and Compression Compared

Concussion is unconsciousness *immediately* following a 'shaking up' of the brain. The patient recovers consciousness but may be dazed and have a headache before he becomes normal.

Where yellow and purple represent consciousness and unconsciousness respectively an episode of *concussion* could be shown diagrammatically like this:

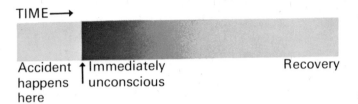

Accident happens here ↑ Immediately unconscious — Recovery

Compression gives unconsciousness which develops *gradually*, the patient moving from awareness, through headache and confusion, into coma.

TIME ⟶

Accident ↑ — Confused — Gradually unconscious

There is no reason why both conditions could not happen from the same accident. A man may recover from concussion and yet bleeding in his skull may be beginning to form an enlarging pressure pool of blood. After a lucid interval, in which he might declare how he feels quite well again, the patient is overtaken by compression. He becomes confused and then comatose. The result would be as if the two diagrams had been superimposed.

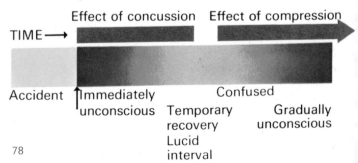

Effect of concussion   Effect of compression

TIME ⟶

Accident ↑ Immediately unconscious   Confused

Temporary recovery
Lucid interval

Gradually unconscious

Beware of rejoicing too soon when a patient, knocked out by a head blow, recovers consciousness. Watch out for the possibility of his worsening.

Beware too of the situation where unconsciousness from compression takes over before the patient has recovered from the unconsciousness of concussion. There is no lucid interval:

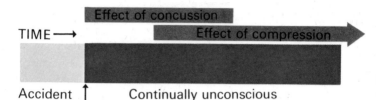

Note that concussion may be accompanied by a fractured skull. Also that fracture of the skull can take place without the bone being significantly displaced and without its pressing on the brain. And remember that it does not need a big blow to cause bleeding inside the skull.

In other words concussion, compression and fracture are separate entities which may or may not occur from the same accident. For the safety of your patient always assume (until proved otherwise) that they co-exist.

Treatment of Head Injuries

This is exactly as for unconsciousness (page 69). Even if the patient is conscious it is a wise precaution to keep him in the recovery position. *Ensuring a free air passage for breathing is the first aider's immediate and most important single action to protect the patient from death.*

In positioning the patient be extremely careful not to twist the head and neck, lest the neck be already injured.

Look extremely carefully for other injuries. There is a big likelihood that you may find them.

Be meticulous about dressing even the smallest wound of the scalp or forehead; this may protect against infection of a skull fracture or of the brain.

If there is bleeding from nose or ear, lie the patient on the same side as the bleeding to let the blood run clear. Do not put

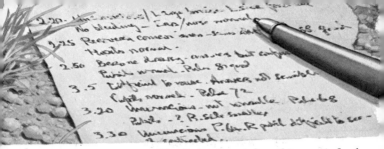

in any plugging since a blood clot dammed up this way is food for microbes and liable to cause infection. Just cover the bleeding organ lightly with a clean dressing.

When in charge of the patient for any length of time note and write down at suitable intervals his degree of consciousness, the pulse rate and the size of both pupils. If compression is developing your records, even on a scrap of paper torn from a notebook, can point to changes and be a valuable guide to the doctor who takes over. The degree of consciousness in the first few minutes after the blow is essential information.

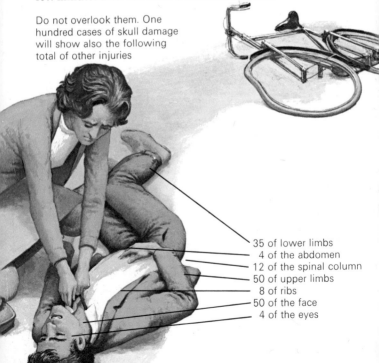

Do not overlook them. One hundred cases of skull damage will show also the following total of other injuries

35 of lower limbs
4 of the abdomen
12 of the spinal column
50 of upper limbs
8 of ribs
50 of the face
4 of the eyes

If you have to keep watch on a head injury patient who has now gone to sleep normally, yours is the problem of deciding whether his continued unconsciousness is natural sleep or developing coma. There is no help for it; you will have to wake him half hourly to make sure his mind is clear. He may not appreciate this. If his speech and directness at each waking are reassuring, his choice of words may need sympathetic understanding.

Postscript on Wounds and Injuries

Finding one wound does not exclude the presence of another. Never treat one without looking for its less obvious companions. Never assume that one swollen area means but one part damaged. A blow to the head can also be a blow to the neck; the fractured pelvis might be associated with internal injuries of the abdomen or chest; the motorist's smashed knee or ankle suggests as well a fracture in hip or foot from impact forces travelling along the limb.

Suspect severe internal damage if the victim has received a blow hard enough to imprint on his skin a bruise mark patterned from his clothes.

Do not imagine that unconsciousness always indicates a head injury. Remember that its many possible causes include lack of oxygen. Always and immediately ask yourself of the unconscious patient: 'Is he breathing or does he need artificial respiration?' and 'Can he breathe or is there some obstruction to the passage of air?'

Pattern bruising. The tell-tale marks of deeper damage

BREATHING FOR LIFE

For life all parts of the body 'burn' oxygen, converting it to carbon dioxide. This last must be got rid of as its accumulation would be very harmful. These processes depend on breathing in the lungs and of blood circulation through the heart beat:

1. *The chest size increases*, achieved mainly by

   a) enlarging the chest size all round by the pull of muscles between adjoining ribs (see illustration, page 106).

   b) increasing the top to bottom dimension of the chest by the flattening down of the dome shaped muscle we call the diaphragm or midriff; shelf-like, it partitions off the lower end of the chest from the upper part of the abdomen.

2. *Air is drawn in* as the chest expands. Passing through the nose and mouth, down the windpipe and the many branching air tubes it finally reaches clusters of the microscopically small air sacs of the lungs. A large part (one fifth) of the air consists of oxygen.

3. *Gases are exchanged at the air sacs.* Blood vessels surround each minute air sac. Oxygen passes into the vessels; by dissolving in the blood it becomes available to be carried all over the body. At the same time the unwanted carbon dioxide dissolves out of the blood and enters the sacs as a gas.

4. *The chest decreases in size* as its muscles relax. Air within the lungs is exhaled, and with it the thrown off carbon dioxide passes out. The whole respiratory cycle is now repeated and, as we have already noted (page 22), there are normally about twelve to sixteen such cycles each minute.

5. *The blood is circulating continually*, propelled by the pumping, or 'beating', of the heart – normally about sixty to eighty times a minute. Each beat sends the oxygen rich blood to the body tissues, and the carbon dioxide laden blood back to be replenished at the air sacs of the lungs.

Obstructed Breathing

We must recognise the difference between the cessation of and the obstruction of breathing.

Cessation of breathing. The centres in the brain which control respiration are no longer acting. The patient's chest is not

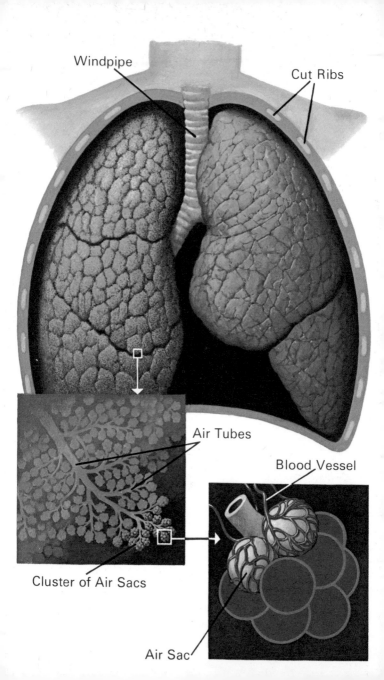

Windpipe

Cut Ribs

Air Tubes

Blood Vessel

Cluster of Air Sacs

Air Sac

moving. He is making no attempts to get air in and out of his lungs. He needs artificial respiration urgently (page 88).

Obstructed breathing. Normal breathing is almost inaudible. Suspect an obstruction when the patient breathes noisily. A quite harmless example is snoring. But in the dangerous type something blocks the passage of air into the lungs. It may be from outside; a plastic bag or cushion over the face, or strangulation at the neck. It may be within the mouth: the tongue's falling back to block the throat (page 68) or the impaction of a toy which a child has been sucking. It could be inside the windpipe: blood or vomit or a large lump of food which had 'gone down the wrong way'. Heavy vapours and smoke may also stifle.

In each case the patient's neck and throat will be making desperate movements to try to shift the obstruction; there will be coughing, or spluttering and choking. Breathing is noisy, and rough, or wet and bubbly. This man does not need artificial respiration; he needs the obstruction removed quickly. (Of course lack of oxygen may eventually so harm his brain that his chest is no longer able to move or his heart to beat spontaneously and by then he has become a case for resuscitation.) Remember that the real victim of air lack is the brain. If the patient recovers after prolonged deprivation he may do so with permanent mental impairment.

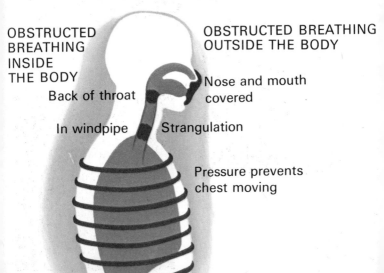

OBSTRUCTED
BREATHING
INSIDE
THE BODY
Back of throat

In windpipe

OBSTRUCTED BREATHING
OUTSIDE THE BODY

Nose and mouth
covered

Strangulation

Pressure prevents
chest moving

Another cause of obstructed breathing is imprisonment of the body under a heavy fall of soil or sand. Even if the patient's face is clear, respiratory movements are prevented by compression around the chest wall.

First Aid

This is obvious: try to remove the cause of the obstruction at once; if necessary follow up with resuscitation.

Tear away any obstruction from mouth and nose.

If the patient is lying down and unconscious the falling back of his tongue may be choking him (page 68). Bend his head back and turn him in the recovery position (page 71).

Open the patient's mouth wide and feel deeply with your finger whether there is anything lodged at the back which you can scoop free.

In cases of hanging support the patient by his legs to relieve the pull; cut the rope and be ready to catch the full weight of the released victim; lay him down; ease the tight band at the neck.

In burial under falls of earth clear the face, chest and abdomen rapidly; be on your guard for possible fractures.

With choking patients interfering is not always wise. It does not need experience to recognise two sorts of choking:

1. The alert, active coughing and spluttering patient whose cough is a healthy reflex to get the obstruction up. Leave him to his resources, but watch closely. You can advise him to breathe very slowly and deeply; this may help to reduce the spasm of the windpipe muscles which grip tightly round the obstructing object.

2. The patient so obstructed that he is becoming blue, limp or unconscious and cannot breathe. A quick attempt to hook out anything from the back of the throat should be made, but may find nothing. Try to dislodge the deeper obstruction with a series of quick hard blows between the shoulder blades, positioning the patient quickly:

   AN ADULT rolled on his side.

   A CHILD held over your forearm or your bent knee, with his head down.

   A SMALL CHILD held (very firmly) upside down by the ankles.

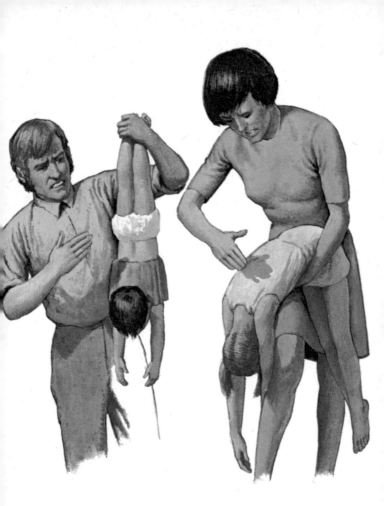

If you succeed you can congratulate yourself. If you have failed or if the patient is still limp and blue *go straight into artificial respiration* and keep at it. Firm slow blowing will sometimes get air past the blockage and will let your patient survive until specialist help comes. The likelihood of your blowing the obstruction object deeper in is a very small one.

RESUSCITATION

In first aid the word 'resuscitation' covers the restoration to life of those who are near death because:

> either their breathing has stopped:
>
> or their heart beat *and* their breathing have stopped.

Please note now – and for ever – four important things:

1. A patient's breathing mechanism can stop but his heart beat may continue yet for a little while. Artificial respiration given in time may save him.

2. If the patient's heart stops so does his breathing. (Though sometimes he may give a few isolated gasps of breath for a short time after.) The resuscitators will have urgently to try to restore both respiration and heart action.

3. There is a dangerous tendency to apply resuscitation to those who have merely collapsed or fainted and whose breathing and circulation are still functioning adequately. It sounds so well afterwards to claim that the 'kiss of life' (a phrase beloved of journalists) was applied, but this may have been utterly inappropriate and even harmful. Do not rush to heart massage and artificial respiration thoughtlessly.

4. On the other hand when these are needed they are needed IMMEDIATELY. You cannot read it up while the patient is lying there. You must learn and practise, and revise repeatedly. Become and REMAIN ready to go into action with instant perfection.

When is Resuscitation Needed?

Breathing and heart beating may cease after:

Suffocation, strangling, choking, through oxygen lack to the vital control centres in the brain.

Drowning. Not only is there oxygen lack. Blood which comes to lungs holding water instead of air undergoes deep chemical and physical changes which harm all the body, and particularly the action of the heart.

Poisoning. Heavy overdoses of certain poisons (strong pain killers or sleeping tablets) may inactivate the life control centres in the brain.

Some gases like carbon *mon*oxide prevent blood from carrying oxygen to the tissues. It is present in escaping unburnt coal gas. It may be found in exhaust fumes of a car; hence the risk of running the engine in a closed garage.

Natural gas (unlike coal gas) has no carbon monoxide in it. But whenever anything burns steadily in small and unventilated quarters the atmosphere loses oxygen and accumulates carbon monoxide.

Electric and Lightning Shocks when the current harms the heart or the nerves controlling chest action.

Some heart attacks where suddenly the beat stops. In a few cases it may be possible to stimulate the heart back into action.

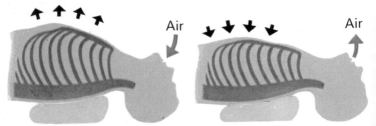

MOUTH TO MOUTH
Blow in   Air escapes

SILVESTER METHOD
Air   Air

ARTIFICIAL RESPIRATION

Modern tests show that by far the most efficient way is for the rescuer to breath directly into the patient's mouth and then let the air flow out naturally between each breath. This is the basis of the Mouth-to-Mouth method and its variations.

There are circumstances, such as a patient's face injuries, which exclude this technique. The first aider then uses one of the chest action imitations, such as the Silvester or the Holger Nielsen (described on page 96).

The Need of Speed

Whatever the method used get the first breaths of air in AT ONCE. Do not think the situation over, or dispose your patient in deliberate and decorous way. Not one second must be wasted. Treat the patient where you find him. (Unless threat of immediate additional danger demands that he be moved).

Whichever method of artificial respiration is used IF THE FIRST FEW BREATHS FAIL TO IMPROVE THE PATIENT'S COLOUR, HE MAY NEED IMMEDIATE HEART MASSAGE. See page 100.

Mouth-to-Mouth Method

This the method of choice.

The step-by-step description below is artificial. These actions are done rapidly, merging smoothly into one man-oeuvre.

1. *The patient is turned on his back.*
2. *His head is tilted back as far as possible.* This is further than you think, and should result in the nostrils looking almost directly upwards. This keeps the tongue from blocking the airway (page 68).

   Cup one hand under the patient's neck, which you lift slightly. Put the heel and palm of the other hand on his forehead, so that your forefinger and thumb reach his nose. Lever the head back.
3. *Pinch the nose shut* at its lowest end with forefinger and thumb. (This, by the way, gives you an additional grip to help pull the head back.)
4. *Make sure the patient's mouth is open.* If it is not, shift the hand from under his neck to the front and lower part of his jaw and pull it to open his mouth. At the same time you can push the jaw to jut forwards as this increases the size of the airway at the back of the throat.

   Take care to keep your finger tips from the patient's lips (for you are about to bring your own mouth down here) and also to keep the edge of your hand from pressing against his neck and windpipe.
5. *If necessary clear the mouth.* Someone rescued from the river, for instance, may have the back of the throat blocked by weeds or mud. In other cases food or a slipped denture

Seal your mouth over
the patient's open
mouth.

may be obstructing. Clearing is done *extremely quickly*; a
forefinger pushed in the opened mouth is swept round in
one fast movement.

6. *Take a deep breath in yourself.*
7. *Seal your wide open mouth over the patient's open mouth.*
   Make sure your lips are firmly in position, over-spreading
   the whole of his mouth.
8. *Breathe into the patient* firmly and fully. Do not make it a
   hard puff; let it be a steady controlled blowing which will

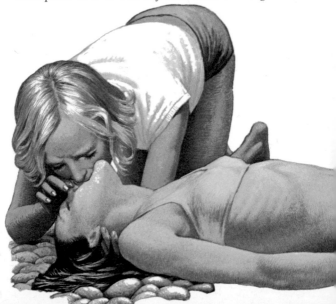

enter the patient's lungs. While you blow watch the patient's chest to make sure that it is rising as his lungs fill up with your air.

9. *Lift your mouth off and let the patient's chest empty* naturally. Turn your head sideways as you do this. Your cheek can feel the air coming out; your ear can hear it; your eyes can confirm that the risen chest is now sinking. At the same time take in a good breath so that as soon as the patient's chest has emptied you can:

10. *Repeat stages 7, 8 and 9 as long as is necessary.* You may find that you get a timing of about 12 breaths a minute. But be guided by the natural movements of the chest and by the amount of air you are managing to get in and out of it.

The Important Extras

Now that the basics have been mastered, finer points of technique have yet to be learnt.

Give the first five breaths rapidly to replenish the patient's blood with oxygen without timing yourself by the sinking of the chest. After this the necessary amount of oxygen can be maintained by the steady breathing described in stages 8 and 9 above. Do not, through a sense of urgency, go on blowing in at speed; such continued deep panting may make you, his rescuer, feel ill and even faint.

If you have to interrupt your artificial respiration, even briefly, resume with the five quick breaths.

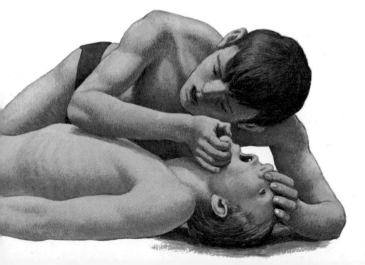

Watch the chest constantly. If it does not rise well as you breathe into the patient check your technique.

Beware of blowing harder than necessary. Aim for the natural rise (and subsequent fall) of the chest. Hard blowing may damage the lungs. It may irritate the stomach and cause the patient to vomit, or it may send air into the stomach as well as into the lungs.

If the patient vomits, quickly turn his head to one side and let the vomit escape. Speedily clean out any which remains in his mouth. Then resume artificial respiration with five quick breaths at first.

If the abdomen becomes distended the stomach probably has filled with air. This could harm by pressure changes on the heart and diaphragm and could also handicap the air entry into the lungs. If you see excessive bulging at the stomach press briefly and gently over this to coax air up and out – but be prepared to deal with any vomit or, in drowning cases, swallowed water coming up as well.

Blocking the nose can be done not only by pinching it, but also by pressing your cheek against the nostrils as your mouth lies on the patient's.

The Mouth-to-Nose Method. You may not be able to use the patient's mouth if it will not open, or has an intractable blockage. Then use the fingers on one hand to keep the patient's lips firmly shut and breathe into him with your mouth sealed round his nostrils.

The Mouth-to-Mouth and Nose Method. With a child, especially a baby, your lips should cover and seal round both

Seal your mouth over a child's mouth and nose

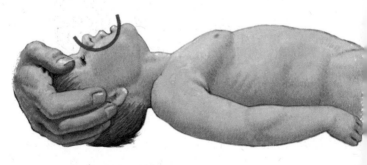

Are your lips fully sealed right round the patient's mouth?

Is the jaw pushed forward with the mouth open?

Are the back of the throat and the windpipe clear?

Is the nose properly pinched shut low down?

Are you still keeping the head bent back as far as possible?

Points to bear in mind

his mouth and his nose. Remember that you blow only just hard enough to get a natural chest expansion. Do not let your adult strength harm the child's lungs; small babies need only quite gentle puffs. You may find that you get a faster in-and-out rate per minute with the young: about 20 in children and about 40 in small babies.

Artificial Respiration is carried out until a doctor tells you to stop because the patient is dead or until the patient breathes for himself. If alone with the patient you have a difficult responsibility, but you must carry on – and shout for help between breaths.

Use helpers to send urgent messages for ambulance or medical help. Let them attend to important secondary features such as loosening tight clothes (belt, braces, collar, corsets) and covering with blankets. Do not interrupt your work unless you have someone alongside ready and instructed to take over as you stop. Continue while the patient is moved onto a stretcher or into the ambulance (which will probably have oxygen apparatus). 'Mouth-to-mouth' can be given under all sorts of unusual circumstances; to a linesman strapped up a telegraph pole, to the child being carried, to the beached bather whose face is just out of water and even to the bather far from shore and out of his depth provided the rescuer is a strong swimmer.

When the patient begins to breathe for himself it may be feebly and barely discernible against your work, or in sudden irregular gasps. Give him a chance to do his own spontaneous breathing now, but small additional breaths from you may be needed to help at this time. Once you are satisfied that his own breathing is good, turn him into the recovery position (page 71). Remain close by and watching lest he suddenly fail and you have to take over again. However well the patient appears to have recoved he must be sent to hospital.

Some Objections Answered

Would training not be very embarrassing? The use of life-like manikins on which to work solves this problem in organised first aid courses. All are urged to follow courses (page 156). In any case there is every moral and human justification for practising on co-operative relatives, friends or fellow students. The very next day might bring urgent need. One piece of advice: let he who plays the part of the patient be as relaxed as he can, for if he tenses up the 'rescuer's' part becomes very difficult.

Could not 'mouth-to-mouth' be most unpleasant? For whom? Not for the resuscitated. In the life-saving business social or aesthetic niceties take second place. Veritable patients are all too often vastly different from the neat manikin. They may be covered in dirt or vomit, and may look dreadful. A true first-aider overcomes his repugnance and goes straight in to help.

A handkerchief stretched out between the two mouths is often suggested, but it is likely to become a sodden mess and a shifting encumbrance. Gadgets for avoiding direct contact with the patient can be timewasters. The immediate, the very first, apparatus is the human one.

What is the good of giving 'second-hand' air? It is true that exhaled air from the first-aider carries carbon dioxide and is poorer in oxygen than fresh air. However, the first part of the

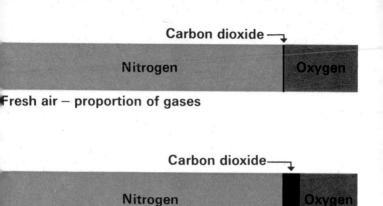

Fresh air – proportion of gases

Air breathed out of lungs

air passing from the rescuer to rescued is that from the rescuer's mouth and windpipe – air which has not been down to the lung sacks and is therefore unchanged. But even that air from the deepest part of the lungs still carries plenty of oxygen and the amount of carbon dioxide it brings with it is too small to harm the patient.

Why not drain water out of a drowned man's lungs? Time-consuming attempts to do so by tipping him up would fail (though it might produce a flow from windpipe, stomach and gullet). Any water left deep in the lungs would remain held by the minute spongy structure of the air sacs.

The urgent thing is to get air in. Correctly applied artificial respiration will bubble air successfully past any fluid which might still lie in the windpipe.

Which takes priority – stopping bleeding or starting breathing? In fact this problem is hardly likely to arise. The non-breather will probably be a non-bleeder. His circulation will be in so poor a way, with so low a blood pressure, that bleeding will have slowed or stopped spontaneously.

Maybe bleeding will show as he recovers – a testimony to your success which may daunt you. By now however you will have the patient sufficiently 'aerated' to allow you to attend to bleeding as well. Also with luck someone will be at hand to help you.

Alternative Methods

It may happen that the patient's face is so badly injured (or even is believed to carry a potent poison) that the first aider should not use his mouth on it. He must then use outer manipulation to expand and contract the patient's chest. The two methods described below are not as effective as the mouth-to-mouth (or to-nose) way which is the first choice whenever possible. But they are excellent alternatives when needs must.

Holger Nielsen Method

This is named after the Danish army officer who introduced it in 1932.

1. *Check that the patient's mouth is clear* (as described on page 89). Be quick.
2. *Turn him on his front.*
3. *Position his head and hands.* The head is turned sideways to let one cheek lie on a 'cushion' of his two hands resting on each other. His mouth and nose must be clear of being obstructed by the ground and his mouth ought to tilt a little downwards (to allow any fluid to drain out).
4. *Kneel in front of him*, one knee near his forehead and the foot of the other leg by his elbow.
5. *Put you hands flat over his upper back*: their 'heels' are at the level of a line joining his armpits; the fingers are spread out over his ribs with your thumbs just touching each other.
6. *Rock forwards* until your arms, which you must keep quite straight, are vertical – and no further. Let the weight of your overhanging body be the acting force; do not shove his ribs. Thus you smoothly compress his chest, driving air from his lungs.
7. *Rock backwards and reposition your hands.* Immediately you begin to rock back slide your hands past his armpits and along his upper arms to grasp them firmly just before you reach his elbows. Continue the rock until your own body is vertical – no further. You will find that your hold on the patient will have lifted his elbows a little way off the ground and so expanded the chest, drawing air into the lungs.
8. *Drop the elbows* and immediately go back to stage 5.

You now repeat stages 5 to 8 smoothly and rhythmically. The cycle takes some six seconds.

Common errors are acting jerkily, waiting too long in the backwards rock to get your hands near the patient's elbows and then pulling his elbows up sharply instead of letting them be drawn up smoothly.

Attention will also be given to loosening tight clothing at the neck and chest, and to covering the patient with coats and blankets.

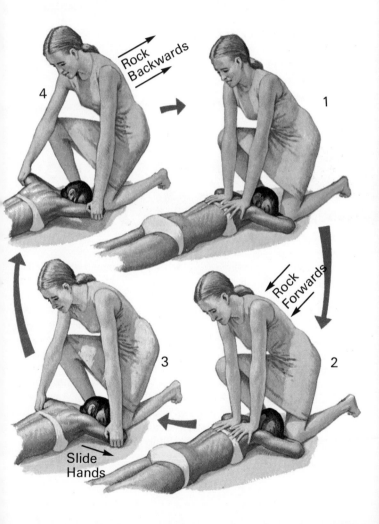

The Silvester Method

The English physician Henry Silvester described this method in 1861. By keeping the patient on his back it will allow heart massage to be done (see page 100). But it needs a cushion under the patient's shoulders to ensure the head's bending back for a clear airway.

1. *Lie the patient on his back rapidly* on a firm surface. A soft mattress will not do.
2. *Raise his shoulders by putting a pack beneath them.* Thus the head bends back as far as possible and the tongue will not block the throat (below). Cushions, folded towels, blankets or coats can be used, but they must be placed as quickly as possible. (A common mistake is to put the pack under the neck instead of under the shoulders.)

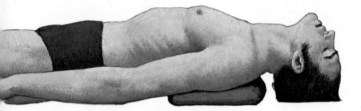

3. *Kneel at the patient's head* with your knees touching his forehead. This is right for a patient about your own size. For a child it might be wise to kneel a little further back. (Some advise having the patient's head between your knees, but you may find this brings you too far forward for balance and control in the movements which are to follow. Practise on different volunteers and find out for yourself.)
4. *Check that his mouth is clear* as described on page 89.
5. *Grasping his wrists bring your hands alongside each other over the lower part of his chest and rock forwards.* Keep your arms straight; the weight of your body will exert the pressure needed to drive air out of the lungs. Do not thrust down jerkily with your arms. For children much less pressure is used than for adults. One can sense the effort needed to compress the chest without crushing it.

Make sure of the position of the hands on the patient's chest. Too high will have but a feeble effect on the lungs. Too low will merely press on the stomach.

6. *Now sweep back the patient's wrists up and out and then down.* Rock back onto your heels as you do this. Be sure that your patient's arms describe a wide arc, with his hands coming down towards the floor alongside you. It is this big swing which expands his chest and draws air into his lungs.

7. *Repeat stages 6 and 7 smoothly and rhythmically.* Let each press-and-stretch take about five seconds (12 breaths a minute). Practise with a watch in front of you.

8. *Keep a constant check that the patient's mouth is clear* and that his head remains fully bent back. If fluid (blood, vomit, water) fills the mouth let it flow out by turning the head to one side. Let anyone helping you attend to this.

Attention will also be given to loosening tight clothing at the neck and chest, and to covering the patient with coats or blankets.

HEART MASSAGE

Heart massage attempts to stimulate back into action a heart which suddenly has become motionless or is quivering so weakly that it is no longer pumping blood round the body.

When the patient's breathing has stopped oxygen lack gives him a blue-tinged pallor. Your immediate duty is to get air into him. After the first five breaths of efficient artificial respiration, as oxygen is distributed by the circulating blood, his colour should markedly improve. However if the heart's pumping has stopped there is no circulation and no oxygen will get through to the tissues. The patient's dreadful colour remains unchanged.

There are signs to help the first aider here: IF AFTER THE FIRST FIVE BREATHS OF ARTIFICIAL RESPIRATION THE PATIENT STILL HAS: DEATH-LIKE PALLOR, ABSENT PULSE, WIDELY-DILATED PUPILS, SUSPECT THAT HIS HEART IS NOT WORKING. AT THE SAME TIME AS ARTI-FICIAL RESPIRATION, EXPERT HEART MASSAGE IS REQUIRED.

Some important points in this statement must be analysed. *The death-like pallor* is blue or grey-tinged. There is the mis-leading exception of poisoning by carbon *mon*oxide, as in coal gas or car exhaust fumes, which may produce chemical changes giving the skin a cherry-pink colour.

The absent pulse is best tested for not by the ear or wrist

Feeling the pulse in the neck

when doing artificial respiration, but on one of the big arteries which runs up either side of the neck. Feel for it with two fingers in the outer and upper part of the neck, along a line pointing towards the angle of the jaw and the ear. (Never try to feel for both at the same time; with inexpert pressure this could temporarily block circulation to a large part of the head; anyway your other hand would be better employed controlling the position of the head.) Examining a pulse does need a little experience and students must practise repeatedly so as to be well prepared if the emergency arises.

Widely dilated pupils (the central dark circles of the eyes) show when the heart has stopped beating. They should contract back to normal size again as both breathing and circulation are restored.

None of these features is absolutely accurate. The degree of the changes and the time for them to occur can vary. Do not, for instance, delay heart massage if you are confident it is needed just because the pupils are not yet widely dilated.

If heart massage is needed artificial respiration is also required. Often artificial respiration is called for without the need of heart massage. But heart massage itself is never given alone. The rule for the first aider is that whenever the heart beating has stopped so has breathing; he must re-activate both.

A man whose heart has stopped, who is unconscious, pulseless and ashen-coloured, may for a brief while yet make an occasional gasping breath.

Finally – and this is just as important: *Heart massage needs expert knowledge.* The student must learn from experienced instructors. He should practise under their supervision. He should understand too that *it can be very harmful to give heart massage when the heart still beats* and is not in need of assistance. (Full practice therefore must be on manikins.)

Why Heart Massage Works

There is a misconception that the heart is entirely on the left of the chest. It lies behind the breastbone, but shifted towards the left side. If the breastbone is sufficiently depressed it pushes down against the front of the heart.

This tends to displace the heart backwards towards the backbone. Because the backbone is large and rigid the heart is

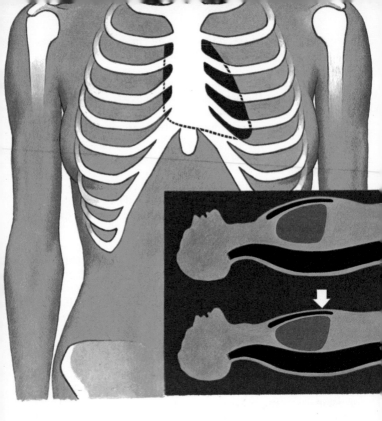

now compressed between two firm surfaces. The blood it contains is forced out into those large blood vessels which form the threshold of the circulation.

Releasing the pressure allows the heart and chest to resume their normal size and shape. Repeating the manoeuvre regularly is now artificially giving the heart a beat which makes it pump blood round the body again.

How to Give Heart Massage

It must be done with great rapidity and smoothness as soon as it is clear that the heart is not beating. Once the heart has stopped nature allows only about four minutes for successful re-activation to be begun. A brain which has been deprived of circulating blood for longer may be irretrievably damaged.

1. *Give three firm slaps over the lower half of the breastbone.* Sometimes this simple action starts the heart beat. If it does not succeed at once:

2. *The patient must be on a hard surface on his back,* with the head bent back in position as for artificial respiration. It would be a waste to try heart massage if the patient is lying on something soft and yielding like a mattress.

3. *Elevate the legs vertically* and keep them propped this way if you possibly can. The return of blood by gravity to the heart may help to stimulate the beat. If you have a helper let him attend to positioning the legs. But do not try this if it is going to delay your next moves.

4. *Kneel alongside the patient. Put the heel of one hand on the lower half of the breastbone and the heel of the second hand on top of the first.* Do not use the lowest part of the breastbone; by leaving the last inch clear you reduce the risk of pressing too low and of damaging the liver, the stomach or other organs. *Keep your fingers and palm off the chest.* Only the *heel* of *one* hand touches the patient. This reduces the risk of spreading the pressure round the chest and of cracking ribs.

5. *Press the breastbone down* by rocking your body forwards and keeping your arms straight. Do not lunge at the patient's chest with a jerk of the arms. Let the effect be a firm thrust rather than a sudden jolt. (The breastbone may sink a couple of inches under pressure. This is quite normal.)

6. *Relax the pressure* by rocking your body back a little and let the breastbone rise spontaneously to its normal state. But keep your hands in position.

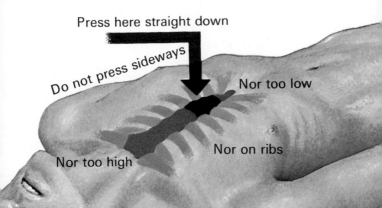

Press here straight down

Do not press sideways

Nor too low

Nor on ribs

Nor too high

7. *Repeat the pressure once a second.* Practise with a watch. The common error is that of going much too fast.

These details are for adults. Children have faster heart beats and more fragile bodies. A baby has a relatively large liver which could be hurt if too much pressure were given too low down.

IN SMALL CHILDREN: *increase the rate* to eighty a minute. *Reduce the pressure* by using one hand only.

IN BABIES: *increase the rate* to a hundred a minute. *Reduce the pressure* by pushing with two fingers instead of rocking over your hand. *Raise the point on which you push* to the middle of the breastbone. This reduces the risk of hurting the liver which in babies is specially large and vulnerable.

8. *Alternate artificial respiration with heart massage.* Both must be done, but in turn, for otherwise the chest actions would contradict one another.

IF YOU ARE ALONE 15 heart pressures alternate with 2 *rapid* breaths of artificial respiration. This is not an easy task but it is a perfectly possible one.

IF YOU HAVE HELP one of you does 5 pressures and then lets the other give one long breath of respiration.

These heart and lung actions must take their turns smoothly, immediately one after the other.

The patient's colour should now improve and his pupils

BY ONESELF

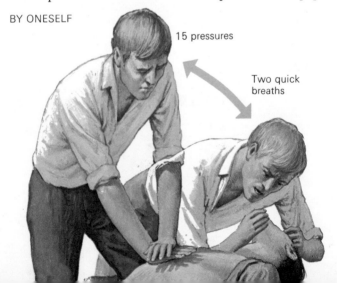

15 pressures

Two quick breaths

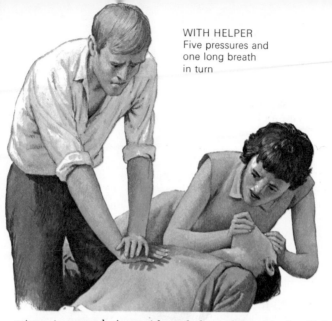

WITH HELPER
Five pressures and
one long breath
in turn

return to normal size; with each beat the pulse should be palpable. Continue until the patient's own heart beat and pulse have returned spontaneously (feel for this in the neck every two or three minutes during one of the breaths of artificial respiration). You will then probably have to continue giving artificial respiration. Watch carefully lest the beat cease again. Resuscitation efforts must continue until the patient is handed over to medical experts. There are recorded cases of several hours' work having successfully brought a patient back to life.

One must face the fact that massage carries some risk of damage to ribs or abdominal organs, especially if done clumsily and especially on the very old and very young. Since the alternative may be death this risk is justifiable.

And Still More Practice

Get familiar with the feel of the breastbone and the position and movements to be taken. Practise everything *except the pressure itself* upon friends and relatives. The pressure is reserved for a manikin or for the real emergency.

INJURIES OF LUNGS AND CHEST

Though there are different types of lung injuries, one first aid approach (page 110) can be used for all.

Severe Bleeding

Coughed up blood is mixed with air and therefore frothy and bright red. This may happen after a blow on the chest wall, a penetrating wound or a blast injury. Occasionally it is due to disease in the lungs.

When a patient lies on his uninjured side, blood coughed up from the damaged lung can overspill at the branching of the windpipe into the side of the healthy lung. To prevent this keep the patient lying on or towards the injured side.

A blow may cause bleeding which remains hidden in the chest cavity. Blood accumulates and compresses the lung, preventing it from expanding properly to draw in air. The compression is minimised if the patient is sitting up.

Open Wounds

We may hear air sucked through a wound flap which acts as a valve preventing air passing out again. This air generally

NORMAL BREATHING

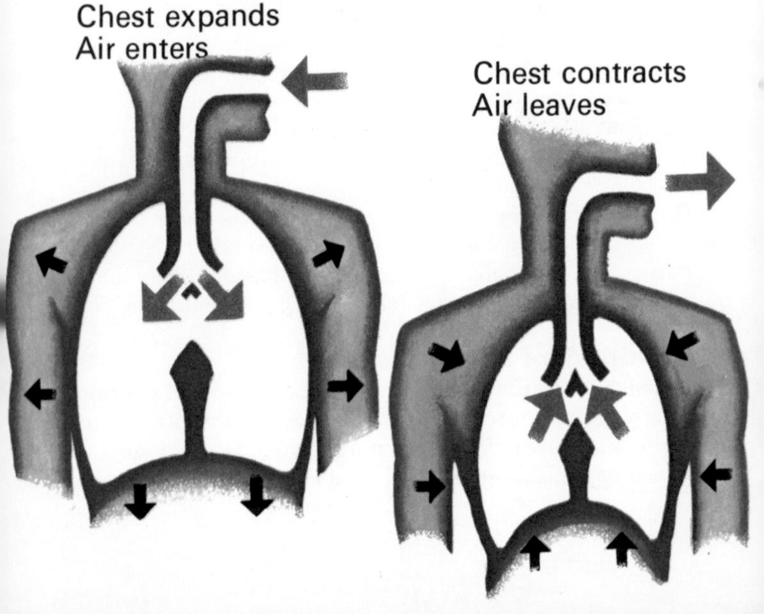

Chest expands
Air enters

Chest contracts
Air leaves

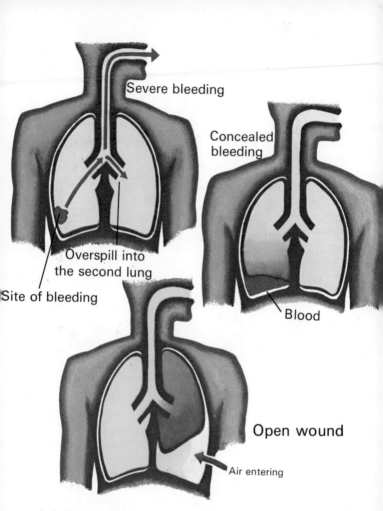

Severe bleeding

Concealed bleeding

Overspill into
the second lung

Site of bleeding

Blood

Open wound

Air entering

spreads between the lung coverings and the chest wall, compressing the lung out of action. It is urgently necessary to cover and close the wound.

Crushed Chest (Stove-in-Chest)

A crushed chest wall – typical of accidents where unbelted car drivers have been thrown against the steering wheel – may

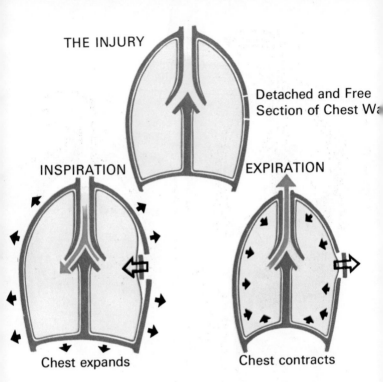

THE INJURY

Detached and Free
Section of Chest Wa

INSPIRATION

EXPIRATION

Chest expands

Chest contracts

fracture ribs extensively. The injured segment, with its detached rib fragments, is independent of the rest of the chest wall; it is free and unstable, no longer obeying the normal force of muscles.

During inspiration the pull of air filling the undamaged lung sucks in this free segment which will sink instead of expanding like the rest of the chest. Conversely at expiration it is bulged forward by the push of the air being breathed out, while the undamaged part of the chest contracts in the usual way.

There are several consequences. Since the damaged chest wall is pulled inwards during inspiration, the lung here can no longer fill up with air. Then, during expiration, the way this segment is pushed forwards prevents the air inside the lung being squeezed out through the air tubes. These defici-

Positioning the chest injury: propped to one side.

encies make it difficult or impossible for the patient to inhale fresh air or to exhale used up air effectively. Nor is he easily able to cough away blood or other obstructions in his air passages.

First Aid

The patient may be coughing up blood and be blue from lack of air. Pain and difficulty in breathing can be eased by the sitting position. Lying down with a damaged lung may be very distressing.

KEEP THE AIRWAY CLEAR. Sweep the mouth rapidly with your finger to clear away blood or vomit, loose teeth or dentures.

CLOSE UP ANY WOUND AT ONCE. Pinch its edges very firmly together or place your whole hand over it. Then plug it with a pad of dressings, handkerchiefs, towels or even part of the patient's clothing. Take great care that whatever you use is bulky and extends well beyond the wound. Now keep it in position by firm and wide bandaging or (better) by overlapping strips of wide adhesive strapping.

IMMOBILISE ANY LARGE UNSTABLE SEGMENT OF A CRUSHED CHEST WALL. Recognise this by its wrong-way-round moving in with inspiration and out with expiration. Your whole hand presses the segment in and fixes it at once as a temporary measure. Now strap or bandage on firmly a thick pad made to fit the area, or even the patient's own forearm as emergency splint. These heroic measures are better than letting the segment move. Such pressure not only controls the abnormal movement, but also relieves pain.

POSITION THE PATIENT half sitting and leaning over to the injured side, if that is known. But keep his weight off any possible fracture. Bank with pillows, folded coats or blankets. This position is a compromise between lying him down (to prevent shock and to let fluid drain from the mouth) and sitting him up (which makes it much easier for him to breathe).

If the patient is unconscious have him lying down in the recovery position (page 71) on the injured side, but avoid pressure on the injury itself. If possible raise the foot of the bed or stretcher some 12 inches.

GET THE PATIENT TO HOSPITAL QUICKLY.

ELECTRIC SHOCK

The current can be compared to a flow of water. The hurt to a man hit by water from a hose pipe depends less on the rate at which the water flows than on the strength of the jet. Similarly with electricity, voltage is a major factor. The higher the voltage the greater the immediate threat to life. Other factors count too: the length of time the current flows in the body or its ease of flow through moist skin or from metal contacts. Water and metal have low resistance to electricity and are good conductors.

Current can be *direct*: constantly flowing in the same direction (like the water of a river). We find this in electricity from batteries or in electrified rails. Current also can be *alternating*, repeatedly changing its direction of flow (like waves created in some washing machines). This is the type for most industrial and domestic circuits. The rate of alternation, the 'frequency', is usually about fifty per second. For the human body this is a bit of bad luck since this frequency is the most dangerous to human nerve and muscle.

Electricity stimulates muscles to contract either as it enters the body (touching or switching on a live point) or when the current is broken (pulling away from or switching off the live point). In between, while the current is flowing steadily, it does not contract muscles (though it can burn the tissues through which it passes). Alternating current, with its constant change of direction, has the effect of being switched on and off fifty times a second, so keeping the muscles constantly contracted. A housewife who picks up the live handle of a faulty electric kettle may have her fist forcibly closed; the contracting muscle will not let her release the lethal handle.

From its point of entry electricity takes the easiest path in the body to an exit point of contact with earth or a good conductor like a metal pipe leading to the earth. Since wet skin is so dangerously efficient a conductor electric apparatus for sinks or bathrooms should be out of reach. Wearing dry insulating footwear or standing on an insulating mat is part of the correct approach to electrical equipment.

Even though the burn mark at the point of contact may be small, the current can spread widely through the body. It causes clotting within the blood vessels in its path, cutting off blood supply to the tissues. Injuring brain and nerves, it can cause paralysis including loss of power of the chest wall and diaphragm so that breathing ceases. The heart muscle may stop beating. These calamities are likely when the current passes through the hands and arms into the chest.

Electricity may kill instantly. Or the victim may be knocked unconscious at once by the shock. Sometimes he feels as if he had been given a very heavy blow. In minor cases he may appear only slightly shaken at the time, but there is a risk that later he becomes very distressed and agitated or unconscious.

First Aid

1. *Release the patient from the current.* Do not touch him yourself or you, too, may receive the shock. *Switch off the current immediately* if you can. All too often this, the simplest and most efficient act, is overlooked. If the switch to be flicked off or the plug to be pulled out cannot be reached try rapidly to *disconnect the patient from the contact.* Pull the insulated cord and try to wrench the plug from its socket or the faulty apparatus from the patient. An alternative is to knock or pull the patient, or the apparatus, with something dry and insulating. A coat can be fast folded into a pad with which to push. Pulling can be done with a walking stick hooked into a limb or armpit, or by a rope or pole or a light chair. (But beware of umbrellas with their metal shafts.) As a last resort quick kicking with dry footwear can be tried; any current entering the rescuer will probably flow straight to earth and not reach his heart or other vital areas.

2. *Resuscitation is often needed.* This is *the* first aid priority and must be given immediately to those who appear dead or not breathing. Most deaths from electric shock are not immediate, but delayed. Do not accept the appearance of death here; beneath it may lie a life to be salvaged by artificial respiration and heart massage.

    A heart which has suffered electric shock may recover with a dangerously abnormal beat. Get the patient by ambulance to hospital attention urgently. He must be watched, even if he is conscious, lest collapse develops.

    When there are several victims of one incident attend

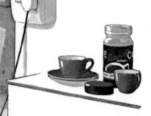

BEST: Turn the switch off or pull the plug out.

NEXT BEST: Pull away by the insulated cord.

OR EVEN: Use available dry non-conductor to knock away the contact.

first to those who are not breathing or who have an imperceptible pulse. Let bystanders, however untrained they may be, help and tell them to imitate your actions as you look after your own patient.

3. *General measures* include attention given to *burns*, which sometimes can be quite extensive from sparks and flashes. Remember that *fractures* may have occurred from falls or from the sudden very powerful muscle contraction due to electricity.

The Problem of Very High Voltages

Rescue by pulling or pushing away from the electrically-live object is possible only for the lower domestic voltage (about 250) or medium voltage (about 500–1000) of industry. The really high voltages (2000–400,000 of power stations or overhead wires) form a very different problem. With such power electricity will leap across gaps into any nearby conducting element, such as a human being – especially if he is carrying metal objects.

Trying to rescue a man still in contact with a very high-voltage conductor may produce two or more victims instead of one. The chances of his survival are too small and the risks in approaching him are too big to justify the attempt. If after contact he had fallen off or been thrown back even using a long pole or dry rope might be dangerous and cause an arc of electricity to flash out to meet one. Would-be rescuers must keep some twenty yards away until the current has been cut off and kept off by the electricity authority.

Lightning

First aid to lightning victims follows exactly the same principles as for those with electric shock. However, there is no question of rescue from the electricity. The current has gone and the patient can be handled at once.

Protection from lightning is highest inside large metal framed buildings or those fitted with lightning conductors, or even inside a metal roofed car. Out in the open follow the advice on the opposite page

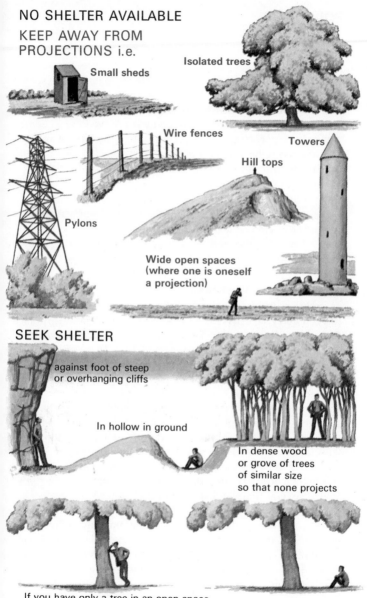

NO SHELTER AVAILABLE
KEEP AWAY FROM PROJECTIONS i.e.

Small sheds

Isolated trees

Wire fences

Towers

Hill tops

Pylons

Wide open spaces
(where one is oneself
a projection)

SEEK SHELTER

against foot of steep
or overhanging cliffs

In hollow in ground

In dense wood
or grove of trees
of similar size
so that none projects

If you have only a tree in an open space
DO NOT lean against it but keep several feet away and **do not touch it**

POISONING

BUT WHAT IS A POISON? Almost anything can be a poison (that is, have a serious harmful effect on the body) if taken in a sufficiently large amount. We can think of *medicines and drugs* such as iron preparations, sleeping tablets or pain killers; some *fruits and plants* like mushrooms and berries; *chemicals* like domestic cleaners, acids, weed killers, petroleum and alcohol.

Not all poisons get into the body by being swallowed. Some can be *injected* through syringes or through the bites of snakes and insects; some, like coal gas can be *breathed in*; some even can be *absorbed through skin*, e.g. agricultural pesticides.

An Orderly System

Fortunately the first-aider's approach to poisoning is not a matter of having to learn a difficult list of antidotes. He can leave that to doctors and be content with remembering a few general straightforward rules.

1. The Patient Must Breathe

Is artificial respiration needed? Prussic acid knocks out the oxygen-carrying cells of the blood. So does coal gas. Morphia-like drugs inhibit the brain's breathing control centre. Pesticides can paralyse muscles, and thus stop respiration.

Is his airway clear? He may be unconscious and therefore need the recovery position (see page 71). He may have been sick and some vomit may choke the windpipe or the back of the throat. (Another possible cause of choking is swelling of the lining to the upper parts of the breathing passages from fumes of corrosive liquids after they have been swallowed. This rare disaster needs a medical man urgently. The most the first aider can do is to apply cold compresses round the neck; this helps a little to reduce the swelling. The compress is a cloth folded several times and soaked in cold water.)

Gas poisoning. Remember that the dangerous carbon *mon-oxide*, colourless and odourless, is present not only in domestic coal gas but also in the exhaust fumes of a petrol engine. A car running in a closed garage (or with a defective exhaust system) can build up a lethal concentration of gas.

Before going in to rescue the victim take a couple of deep

FIRST AID IN POISONING

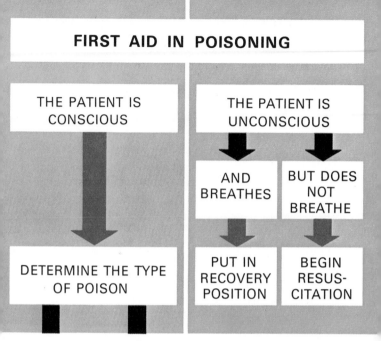

THE PATIENT IS CONSCIOUS

THE PATIENT IS UNCONSCIOUS

AND BREATHES

BUT DOES NOT BREATHE

DETERMINE THE TYPE OF POISON

PUT IN RECOVERY POSITION

BEGIN RESUS-CITATION

AT THIS POINT SEND FOR MEDICAL AID

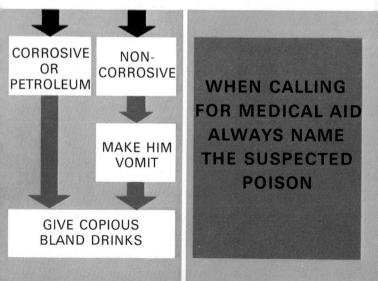

CORROSIVE OR PETROLEUM

NON-CORROSIVE

MAKE HIM VOMIT

WHEN CALLING FOR MEDICAL AID ALWAYS NAME THE SUSPECTED POISON

GIVE COPIOUS BLAND DRINKS

breaths; then hold your breath as long as you can while you go in. Turn off the gas tap (or the engine) and open the windows, but do not spend time on these actions if they prove difficult. Drag the patient out and attend to resuscitation.

2. Identify the Poison

In doubt ask the patient (if he can respond) or bystanders and relatives. Find evidence by smell or in the labels of containers.

At this point decide whether a corrosive or a petroleum product is involved. Their special significance is mentioned below. Corrosives such as strong acids and alkalis leave marks of chemical burning and staining at the lips and mouth of where they have spilled onto skin and clothes. Petroleum preparations have their characteristic smell.

PREVENT POISONING
1. Medicine chest under adult supervision: has child proof lock: sloping top cannot act as shelf. 2. Medicine bottle labels always read before use. 3. Gas taps out of children's reach. 4. Cabinet surfaces free of potential poisons. 5. Cordial bottles used for nothing else. 6. No pill bottles in hand bags. 7. Domestic chemicals out of children's reach. 8. No chemicals on lower shelves.

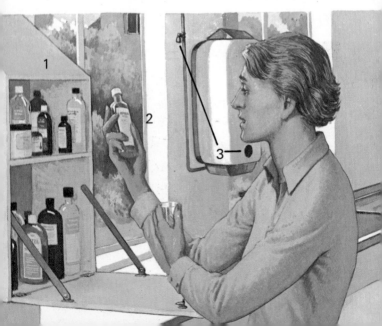

3. Send for Medical Help

At once, and without leaving the patient, delegate someone to speed a message to doctor, ambulance or hospital. The message must be complete (see page 154) and should state the urgency, the suspected poison and a request for advice on any special things to be done before the doctor arrives.

4. Make the Patient Vomit out any Swallowed Poison

This is an important move. What lies in the stomach must be removed before it does more harm. Do not be satisfied with a small vomit; *let the patient be sick many times.*

Give a solution of salt or mustard: two TABLEspoonfuls of salt, or two TEAspoonfuls of mustard, to each tumbler of water which should be just warm if this is easily possible. Repeat this as necessary.

If these are not to hand *tickle the back of the patient's throat*. No light, courteous touch is wanted here; do it boldly with two fingers reaching well back. Small children can be positioned upside down while this is being done.

The patient will not bite if you prevent his teeth from clamping down by shoving a thick wedge of handkerchief or

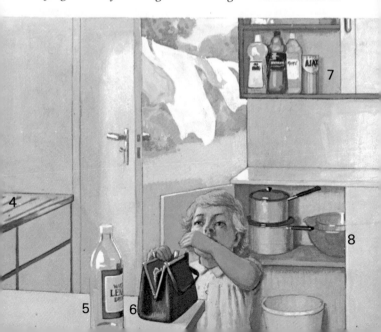

cloth between the jaws at one corner of his mouth. If the patient is co-operative why not let him use his own fingers, provided he does it efficiently?

The result will be far more effective if copious fluid is given. Let the patient take a big drink before each throat-tickling.

VOMITING MUST NOT BE BROUGHT ABOUT:

IF THE PATIENT IS UNCONSCIOUS.

IF THE POISON IS A CORROSIVE. Vomiting is accompanied by violent movements of the stomach. Badly burnt and weakened by the corrosive the stomach wall would rupture during these contortions. In any case the corrosive has already severely hurt the mouth and gullet. Its return journey would but worsen the damage.

IF A VOLATILE PETROL TYPE FLUID HAS BEEN SWALLOWED. The vapours could seriously harm the airways and the lungs as the poison is brought up.

PREVENT POISONING
1. Children warned about poisonous plants. 2. Chemicals kept on high shelves and well labelled. Not to be used while others are in the garden. 3. Manufacturer's instructions followed and protective cover worn when advised. 4. Lock on garden shed. 5. Only harmless material at ground level.

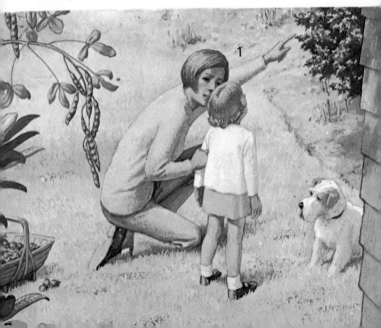

5. Protect the Damaged Stomach by Fluids

Most swallowed poisons do some damage to the stomach's lining. Deal with this by giving drinks which (you hope) will be kept down and not vomited. They are to soothe the stomach and also to dilute any poison still present. The patient drinks copiously, but slowly and carefully – not in big gulps. If he has burnt mouth and lips from a corrosive he may be able to take small painful sips only. Milk is ideal. So is barley water (four times more concentrated than usual). Water will do if nothing else is available. If possible let these be pleasantly tepid. **NOTHING IS GIVEN BY MOUTH IF THE PATIENT IS UNCONSCIOUS. THE PATIENT CANNOT SWALLOW. HE WOULD ALMOST CERTAINLY CHOKE IF GIVEN SOMETHING BY MOUTH.**

6. Measures to Prevent Shock

These come as a matter of course, while awaiting the ambulance. They include lying the patient down, covering him and washing and dressing any skin burns from corrosives.

7. Keep the Patient Closely Observed

Even if he seems to have recovered or to be doing nicely make

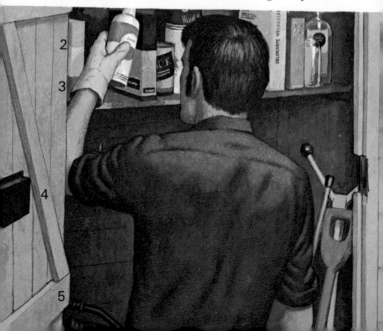

sure someone is constantly alongside him. He may suddenly have a convulsion or vomit; he may lose consciousness, collapse or stop breathing with little or no warning.

If he is a failed suicide case he might suddenly have another attempt at doing away with his life.

8. Keep the Evidence
Leave the medicine bottles, pill boxes or containers as they are. If you are in charge when the ambulance comes see that these go with the patient, as well as a sample of any vomit; they may need testing at the hospital.

Agricultural Poisons
So many different chemicals are used to destroy weeds and pests on the land that no single set of statements can be true for all of them. In man they cause one or more symptoms which could equally belong to many illnesses: headache, flushing, abnormal sweating, excessive thirst, appetite loss, nausea or vomiting, stomach ache, weak and twitching muscles, tightness of the chest, difficulty in breathing, dimmed vision through constricted pupils, coma and convulsions.

Never neglect *any* unusual feelings which appear whilst or within some hours of handling pesticides. For instance consider in danger the worker who develops abmormal tiredness, who suddenly wants to sit and rest or to quench a heavy thirst. If pesticide poisoning is suspected do not wait for definite features to show up before taking action. Early vague symptoms may quickly be overtaken by dangerous severe ones.

Some of these poisons affect nerve or muscle power and so lead to death from failure of breathing and heart beat.

Some are breathed in through nose or lungs and some can be absorbed through the skin where they settle or splash.

Some will harm very rapidly if met in a high concentration but, depending on the amount absorbed, the nature of the chemical and the frequency of exposure, symptoms of poisoning may develop within minutes, hours or days.

First Aid
Make the patient stop work at once and put him at absolute rest. All handling will be gentle. Take him away – on a

stretcher or a board if you can – from any risk of further contamination in the area. Remove clothing which might be contaminated and wash the skin very thoroughly with soap and water. If they have been splashed flush the eyes with gentle copious streams of water. You will take care, of course, not to become contaminated yourself. Where the patient has stopped breathing all this may have to be done while artificial respiration is being given – a situation which will really tax the first-aider's thoughts and actions.

Check whether the container carries any instructions concerning poisoning; let it accompany the patient to the doctor.

Give the conscious patient plenty to drink; sugared water with a pinch of salt helps his energy and puts back into him fluids and chemicals he has lost in the sweat. Naturally if there has been any question of his having swallowed the poison and he is conscious you will make him vomit. (See page 119.)

If he feels abnormally hot cope with this by sponging him with cold water or even by fanning him; keep him in the shade.

PREVENT POISONING. Do not let the bright look of pills fool your children

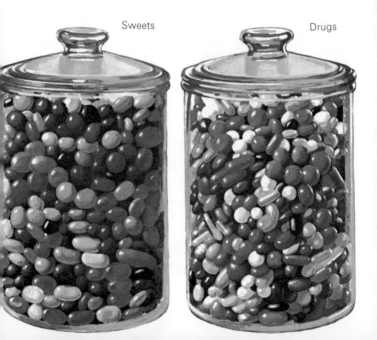

Sweets   Drugs

EFFECTS OF TEMPERATURE CHANGES

Heat Reactions

In excessive heat the body tries to cool itself. Vessels dilate widely in the skin which becomes flushed. Warmth from this extra blood at the surface is shed to the outside air, much as heat is given out from the water inside a domestic radiator. The body is coated with sweat which then evaporates into the air. Change of state from water to vapour uses up a great deal of heat, extracted from the body.

The two main types of thermal crisis, *heat exhaustion* and *heat stroke*, have different causes and effects.

HEAT EXHAUSTION can be met in overheated factories or during the hottest days of summer. It develops gradually, perhaps over several hours or even days. Typical is the patient who has been abnormally energetic, the activity of his muscles creating within him a high temperature which aggravates that of the atmosphere around him.

Reacting normally, he sweats heavily. Sweat is not water alone; it carries with it much salt from the body tissues. Exces-

HEAT EXHAUSTION
Develops gradually especially after unusually hard work. Skin pale, moist, sunken. Pulse fast and feeble. Temperature normal or little raised

sive salt loss causes painful muscle cramps and general weakening. Fluid and salt depleted, the patient is becoming shocked and shows a sunken (and sometimes pale) skin. His pulse is fast but weak. His temperature has been protected by his sweating and may be normal, or not higher than 38°C. (100°F.)

Rest him in bed in a cool atmosphere. Get him to drink a great deal: fruit juices are ideal. But let there be a half-teaspoonful of salt added to each tumblerful of the fluid.

This type of patient is likely to recover well, but seeking medical advice at once is justified.

HEAT STROKE, dangerous and relatively rare, occurs where circumstances prevent the body's protective mechanism from acting. Air temperature may be higher than that of the patient who then gains heat from the atmosphere instead of losing heat into it. The air's humidity may be so high that it cannot take in any more moisture; therefore sweat cannot evaporate from the skin. Or the patient may be wearing many clothes which trap moisture-laden air between the layers. The situation worsens

HEAT STROKE
Develops rapidly in hot, humid, windless air. Irritable, confused or comatose. Skin hot, red dry. Pulse fast, forceful. Temperature very high

if the day is windless, with negligable air changes around the overheated victim.

The resources of the body can break down quite suddenly. Sweating is much reduced or ceases. The patient has a headache and feels tired and irritable. His eyes are inflamed. His pulse is fast and forceful. His skin is burning hot, red and dry. His temperature rises to levels as high as 42°C. (107°F.) He may become confused and even unconscious. Untreated he may die.

The situation is urgent; act rapidly. Rest the patient, if possible on a surface like a canvas camp bed which lets air circulate underneath him. Get his clothes off and sponge him all over with (or put him in a bath of) tepid or cold water. Do not however use ice for that would interfere further with the functioning of skin blood vessels. Fan him, using a machine or waving papers and cloths.

Aim to reduce the temperature to about 39°C. (102°F.) and be content to keep it at that level. To cool him further might cause him to collapse. Take temperature readings every few minutes. This patient needs medical attention urgently.

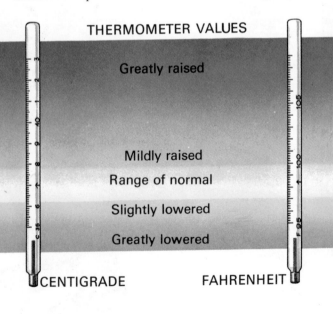

THERMOMETER VALUES

Greatly raised

Mildly raised

Range of normal

Slightly lowered

Greatly lowered

CENTIGRADE   FAHRENHEIT

Cold Reactions
Frostbite

In intense cold blood vessels narrow down so much that the blood supply may be cut off from their area; gangrene is threatened. The skin becomes blanched or blue and is numb. Handle it with great care. Do not rub it – least of all with snow! Do not try to warm it fast.

Remove tight objects like rings, garters, footwear, which might interfere further with the circulation. Remove wet clothes and dry the whole part gently. Cover it, loosely with dry material. Let it warm itself gradually and keep it at rest.

Give the patient warm drinks and get him to a generally warm atmosphere as soon as you can.

Someone who is far from shelter when his hand becomes frostbitten can tuck it under his clothes in his armpit. A dry gloved hand can be cupped over a frostbitten nose, chin or ear lobe.

Exposure

The threat to life from exposure to cold and wet can develop insidiously. Sometimes shivering (the body's attempt to produce heat by muscle action) may suggest that temperature control is failing. The victim slows down mentally and physically; he stumbles and is clumsy; his muscles are cramped and weak and he tends to lag. His character may change: the silent man becomes irrational and talkative; the friendly talker becomes remote and quiet. Within a couple of hours the patient may collapse; in another couple he may die unless treated.

Recognising these features and coping with them at once is essential. Do not try to goad on the stumbling laggard. The patient must be made to stop and should be treated on the spot or be transported by stretcher.

For the conscious patient attempt rapid rewarming. Out in the open he must be protected by a shelter run up from tents, poles or sticks, blankets or coats. Wet clothes are removed as well as any waterproof ones which may be sealing within them the now cold sweat which had formed during recent exertions. Dry the patient quickly and cover him very warmly with blankets or in a sleeping bag. Keep the head and hands well covered too.

The Rescue Blanket is an extremely thin, strong metal foil sheet. Wrapped round the patient it insulates him superbly, reflecting radiant heat from his body back into him. (But he still needs blankets between him and the ground to protect against conductive heat loss.) A Rescue Blanket – 140 cms wide and 210 cms long ($4\frac{1}{2}$ × 7 feet) – folds into a packet which fits into the palm of a hand. It can be bought from camping stores, and should accompany every outdoor expedition.

Further heat can be given by a warm companion under the covering. Give hot sweet drinks such as cocoa.

If you can get the patient to a suitable centre put him in a warm bath at about 43°C. (109°F.). (The baby's bath test: 'bearable by a dipped-in elbow' is quite satisfactory.) Even immersing the patient's arms in basins of hot water helps a little.

Note how for *this* condition we are breaking some of the anti-shock rules. We warm the patient and we give drinks. But we still forbid alcohol (see page 21) and we still must keep his head low (see page 17). He must not be propped or tilted up.

If the patient is unconscious his condition is much more serious and he should be treated as for Hypothermia, that is by gradual (and not by rapid) rewarming.

However *immersion exposure* (i.e. in very cold water) always merits rapid rewarming, whether the victim is conscious or not. Handle the unconscious patient very gently. Beware of artificial respiration and of heart massage as these manipulations may cause an intensely cold – yet still imperceptibly beating – heart to fail. It is rapid rewarming which gives the highest chance of reviving the apparent corpse rescued from an icy sea.

Hypothermia

The word 'hypothermia' (i.e. low temperature) could be applied for any condition of coldness, but is generally used for special cases concerning extremes of age. Babies and elderly people have relatively inefficient temperature defences and may succumb gradually to a cold atmosphere which others could face with only slight discomfort. Too often these frail or defenceless beings sleep in an unheated winter room, with blankets slipping off the bed. In sleep they become chilled and

Hypothermia thermometer

pass into a frozen stupor or into unconsciousness. The situation is worse when they have been taking drugs like some tranquillizers which lower the body temperature, or when babies are so tightly swaddled that they cannot properly move their muscles to create heat.

If the patient's temperature is below 35°C. (95°F.), that is below the lowest point on the range of the normal thermometer, he has passed into hypothermia. The temperature may go as far down as 26°C. (79°F.) before death occurs. A special thermometer is needed to register these ranges.

The patient's consciousness dulls and he becomes slow and dazed and eventually uncomfortable. Pale or blue, his skin is very cold to touch not only at the exposed parts like the face and hands but also at those which are covered. Often it is puffy. Pulse and breathing rates are very slow. (There are exceptions: some babies may show a misleadingly red skin, and near death breathing may become fast).

The first part of treatment is to be aware of the possibility of hypothermia, to recognise it when found and to make an immediate call for medical help.

The way this condition has gradually developed demands that rewarming itself be slow and gradual. Collapse from heart failure is the risk of sudden reheating which widely dilates skin vessels, pooling blood away from the heart and other vital centres. Also the patient's life chemistry had the time to try to adapt slowly to extreme cold; a sudden reversal of circumstances could be fatal.

Put the patient to bed with good, but loose, covering and *without* any extra hot water bottles or electric blankets. But if he is conscious you may give him warm (not hot) drinks to be taken slowly. Let the room itself be warm, at 27 – 30°C. (80 – 85°F.). Get the patient to hospital as soon as you can, or call a doctor immediately.

EMERGENCY DELIVERY

Try to have a doctor or midwife deliver the baby, or to get the patient in labour into hospital in time. But if you have to cope alone do not despair. A fast labour is generally a normal labour and the mother should be told this reassuringly. Following the steps below will probably give a straightforward result even if lacking the finesse of the accomplished obstetrician.

Cleanliness is essential. Scrub your hands and nails thoroughly, under running water if possible.

The first stage of labour usually lasts several hours but may sometimes be disconcertingly brief. The mother feels contractions which dilate the opening of the womb until it is big enough to let the baby pass through. Initially they may be at intervals of about half an hour but then increase in frequency until they come every few minutes. Advise the mother to rest and not to bear down but to relax quietly. A small blood-stained discharge may appear, and is quite normal.

A full bladder impedes the progress of the delivery. At the beginning of labour the mother should be advised to empty her bladder. (Since the birth of a baby is sometimes unpredictably sudden she should use a chamber pot and not the lavatory.)

The second stage lasts until the birth of the child (about one hour but sometimes much less). Now the mother has an urge to 'push' with each contraction. Let her do this, but between contractions she ought to rest and relax.

She lies on her back, and keeps her knees bent up and her feet apart during the contractions. At the beginning of each she takes a deep breath in and out, and then another breath in, which she tries to hold while the contraction lasts. This simple process not only provides fresh oxygen through her blood to the baby, but also helps the mechanics of the womb's contractions.

At some point in the first or second stages there may be a sudden escape of the watery fluid, which has been surrounding the baby. If it alarms the mother reassure her that it is natural.

The birth generally occurs with the baby's head foremost.

PREPARE:
Bed with: 1. Pillow; 2. Blankets; 3. Sheet; 4. Macintosh sheeting.
Table with: 5. Clean basin; 6. Gauze and wool; 7. Clean cover;
8 & 9. Soap and brush; 10 & 11. Scissors and string boiled for 10
minutes in saucepan; 12. Clean towel.
Cot (e.g. small drawer 13.) with: 14. Towels as lining and for
covering the baby (but not to be used as pillow).

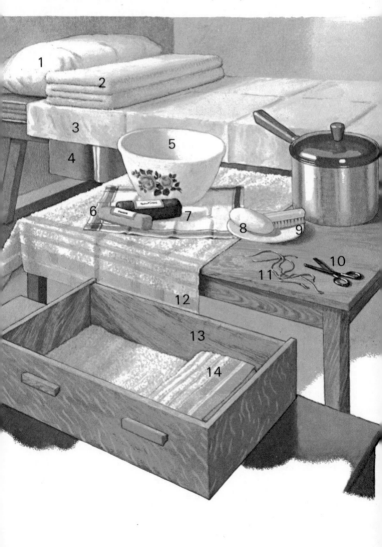

As it emerges the mother is told to pant in quick breaths; this helps to prevent contractions sending the baby out too forcefully. Use your cupped hand over the emerging head not to impede a steady progress but only to guard against a sudden forceful thrust of the head, hurtful to both mother and child. When the head is out do not interfere unless you can see or feel that the umbilical cord is wrapped round its neck. In this case try to loop the cord up and ease it over the head before it is tightened by the advance of the baby in the next contraction.

Support (but don't grasp or pull) the baby's head in the palms of your hands and wait for the next contraction which delivers the shoulders. Now hold its body firmly under its armpits and lift it fully out. Be careful in handling: the baby is wet and slippery. The cord must not be pulled or stretched.

Immediate care of the baby. Hold the baby *firmly* upside down by the ankles to let any fluid drain out of the mouth and nose; wipe these clear with swabs. When it cries lay it close to the mother, on its side with head low, and tuck a towel around it.

If he does not cry within two minutes of birth start artificial respiration gently by the mouth-to-mouth and nose method (see page 92), blowing very gently.

The third stage may last five to twenty minutes. It expels the after-birth (to which the other end of the cord is attached) by further contractions with the mother helping by bearing down as it comes. Keep the after-birth for inspection by the doctor or midwife. If there is much bleeding gently but firmly massage the top of the womb which now can be felt at approximately the level of the navel. The massage stimulates contractions which squeeze shut the bleeding areas of the womb.

Dealing with the cord. If a midwife or doctor is expected shortly, then leave this to the expert. Otherwise ten minutes after the birth of the baby (whether the after-birth has been delivered or not) tie the string round the cord really firmly in two places about 6″ and 8″ from the baby's navel. Unless the tie is very secure the baby may bleed to death once the cord is cut. Cut the cord between the two ties. Put a clean dry dressing over the cut of the end on the baby. Two minutes later inspect this to make sure there is no bleeding. Make a third tie between the existing one on the baby and the navel. Wrap the baby in a

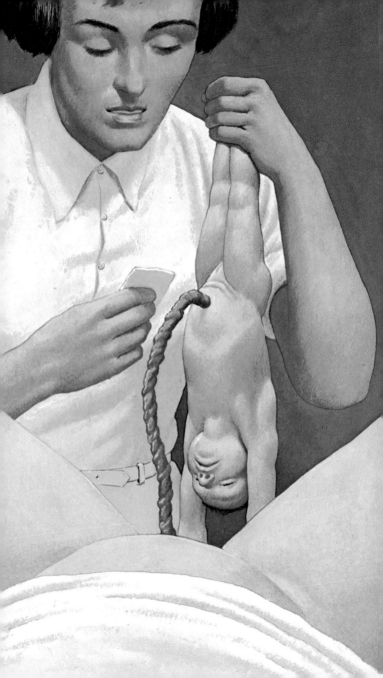

clean blanket or towel and place him in the cot with the head low and to one side.

Care of the mother. Put a sanitary towel in position. Give her warm drinks. Congratulate her and let her rest and sleep if possible.

The Threat of a Miscarriage

If in early pregnancy a woman begins to have vaginal bleeding she may be beginning to miscarry. Even though the amount of blood is small its presence must be heeded as a warning. The risk is greater if she has pains in the abdomen or back.

Tell her to go to bed and remain there until the doctor (whom you will notify) gives his own instructions. Let her keep for the doctor to examine any clots or material she may pass; their appearance could guide him as to what is taking place.

Dealing with the umbilical cord

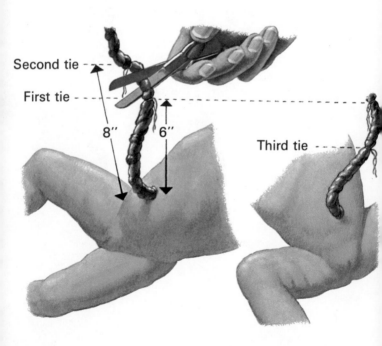

Second tie

First tie

8"

6"

Third tie

MINOR NUISANCES

Strained Muscles

Strains are the overstretching of muscles, with perhaps some of the fibres torn (not to be confused with sprains of joints). Sudden jerking of a limb, or coping with a very heavy weight are likely causes. Strained areas are painful, with reduced or weakened movement. Bruising and swelling may or may not appear according to the depth and extent of the injured muscles.

Essentially treatment consists of resting the muscles. A cold compress (see page 67) can help if it is applied immediately since it reduces the blood flow and therefore limits the swelling and bruising. But there is little point in trying the compress several hours after the injury.

A crepe or an elastic bandage is very useful. The bandage must be applied slightly stretched so that it gives firm support and each turn should overlap the previous one by about two thirds of its width. At the time it is put on the patient must be invited to say if it feels too tight and certainly he should be allowed the option of adjusting it later if it feels too restrictive. Put very tight directly on the skin an elastic bandage can constrict blood vessels and can cause numbness, pallor or swelling of the area beyond it. Joints where main blood ves-

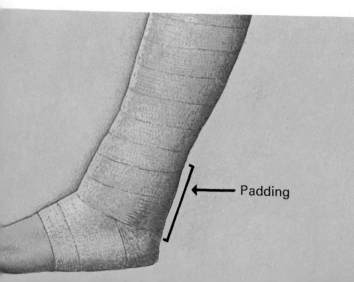

← Padding

sels come close to the surface – the ankle, knee, wrist and elbow should not be covered with an elastic bandage by the first aider unless there is cotton wool padding to buffer the pressure.

Cramped Muscles

Nothing could be simpler than overcoming sudden cramps: stretch the muscles involved as far as they will go. Cramp at the calf can be 'switched off' by straightening the knee and bending the foot upwards at the ankle. For the back of the thigh the same stretching effect can be achieved by pulling the leg well forward and also straightening the knee. Fingers bent in cramp can simply be pressed out straight.

Remember that loss of salt from sweating, vomiting or diarrhoea can be a cause of cramp.

Insect Stings

The immediate irritation and pain of the sting can be greatly eased if an antihistamine cream is applied at once, gently rubbed in. (There are plenty of such creams to choose from and your doctor or chemist can advise which to have in your first aid kit.) If you have not got any cream try immersing the area in cold water or applying a cold compress (see page 67).

Later trouble from a sting – increasing pain and inflammation – developing over the next day or two indicates infection and a doctor's advice would now be needed.

Sometimes the insect leaves his sting behind, projecting from the skin. Pull it out with fine tweezers, but place them near the buried tip of the sting, against the skin; putting them higher may squeeze in any of the sting poison which still remains. (No tweezers to hand? Well cleaned finger nails make an excellent substitute.)

Rarely emergencies arise rapidly from insect stings. Someone who has developed high sensitivity to the sting poison or who is heavily stung by many insects may collapse. He should be treated as for preventing shock. A sting inside the mouth may give so rapid and extensive swelling at the throat that the patient has difficulty breathing past it. Ice to suck or a cold compress (see page 67) at the neck is of some help. In these emergencies immediate medical help is needed.

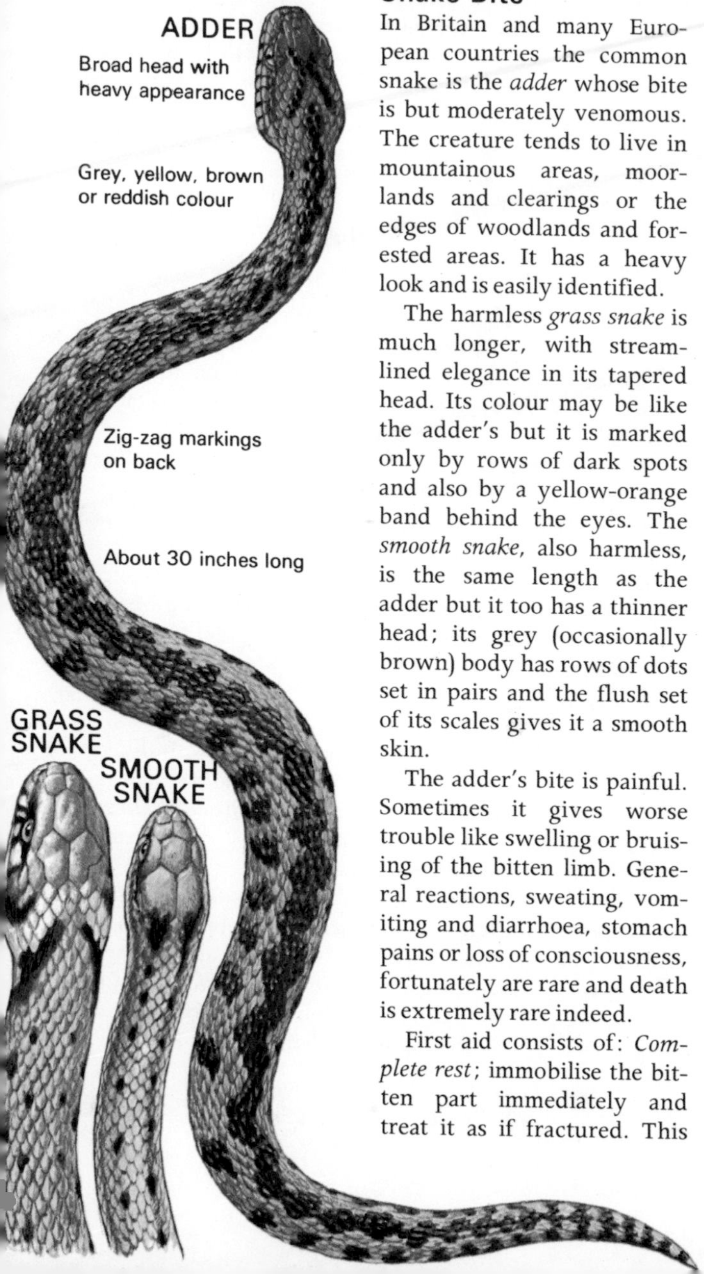

ADDER

Broad head with heavy appearance

Grey, yellow, brown or reddish colour

Zig-zag markings on back

About 30 inches long

GRASS SNAKE

SMOOTH SNAKE

Snake Bite

In Britain and many European countries the common snake is the *adder* whose bite is but moderately venomous. The creature tends to live in mountainous areas, moorlands and clearings or the edges of woodlands and forested areas. It has a heavy look and is easily identified.

The harmless *grass snake* is much longer, with streamlined elegance in its tapered head. Its colour may be like the adder's but it is marked only by rows of dark spots and also by a yellow-orange band behind the eyes. The *smooth snake*, also harmless, is the same length as the adder but it too has a thinner head; its grey (occasionally brown) body has rows of dots set in pairs and the flush set of its scales gives it a smooth skin.

The adder's bite is painful. Sometimes it gives worse trouble like swelling or bruising of the bitten limb. General reactions, sweating, vomiting and diarrhoea, stomach pains or loss of consciousness, fortunately are rare and death is extremely rare indeed.

First aid consists of: *Complete rest*; immobilise the bitten part immediately and treat it as if fractured. This prevents or slows spread of the poison. *Reassurance*; let the patient realise that even for snakes far more poisonous than the adder discomfort and pain are likely to be most he will suffer. *Cover the bite* with a dry dressing. *Relief of pain* by aspirin or paracetamol tablets. *Transport to* hospital quickly and, if possible, lying down. But do not waste time if a stretcher-carrying car is not immediately available.

Please FORGET old-fashioned teaching about washing, sucking or cutting the bite, applying chemical crystals or using a tourniquet.

An Object in the Ear Canal

This is more likely to be a pin, broken matchstick or child's bead than the maligned earwig. Poking about for it carries quite a risk of hurting the ear drum which closes the far end of the canal. So leave the problem to the doctor unless:

1. You can let the object fall out by simply bending the patient's head well to the side,
2. You think the object can float. In that case lie the patient with the ear uppermost and gently pour in a little water to bring the intruder to the surface. Even this simple measure is best left out if the ear hurts or if you believe the ear drum is damaged; water might pass through, carrying infection to deeper structures.

Objects in the Nose

Children are the chief culprits, experimenting with things like beads or beans. The latter tend to absorb fluid and to swell up inside the nose, making the problem more difficult. The object may be forgotten by the child, only to cause a badly smelling discharge from the nose some days later.

Gentle nose blowing (not sniffing – some children do not understand the difference) may help if the object is small and loose. An object which can be easily grasped at the nostril tip presents no difficulty. But do not be tempted to probe for one which is well inside; you may push it in deeper and you may hurt the nose. Let the doctor deal with it.

Removing an object from the eye. The numbers refer to the relevant paragraphs in the text

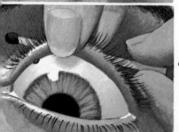

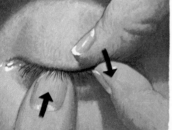

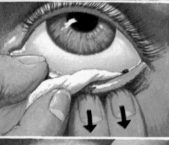

An Object in the Eye

Anything *embedded* in the surface of the eye should be left for the doctor to handle since inexperienced attempts at removal without the right equipment may injure the eyeball. The same veto applies to an object stuck over the coloured ring (iris) or the central dark circle (pupil): these overlie the lens of the eye and scarring would be most damaging. In such cases secure a pad over the eye while awaiting medical help.

Generally the object lies loose under one or other lid and more often than not it is the upper lid.

Wash your hands thoroughly and have by you a piece of cotton wool or the soft fold of a handkerchief; moisten these and shape them into a point with which to touch and lift out the particle.

1. Sometimes the patient can get rid of the trouble by blinking his eye under water.

2. If this does not work or is not possible sit him down in a good light. Stand behind him, with his head resting firmly against your chest.

The patient looks upwards, gently press one or two fingers below the eye, drawing the skin down and so everting the lid. See if you can spot any particle on it; look well into each corner.

3. If this shows nothing let the patient look down while you grasp the upper lid and pull it straight down over the lower lid. Keep the latter slightly and gently pushed upwards. Then let go both lids and hope that the lower one may brush away the object from under the upper. You may need several tries.

4. If the particle still has not moved look for it under the upper lid. Pull this lid upwards and backwards, everted over a match which you press back gently along the lid's 'hinge' while the patient looks down. (It is kinder to have the rounded head of the match against the patient's nose and the square end in your fingers).

Grasp the lid firmly. This is more comfortable for the patient than a light hold which lets the lid slip away.

Blisters

Blisters will form from burns and also (as ill shod hikers can testify) from repeated rubbing and chafing. Do not break the blister as this increases the risk of its infection. A dry dressing is the treatment. However when the blister gets in the way of clothing and activity it should be pierced with careful method.

The blister itself and the surrounding skin are washed with soap and water or with cetrimide solution (see p. 48). A large needle is sterilised either by boiling in water for ten minutes or by holding it in a flame to make it red-hot. Do not then let the needle point touch anything until it pierces the blister.

Puncturing is done at two or more points at the base of the blister. Some fluid will ooze out; the rest can be pressed away by flattening the top with a piece of cotton wool or gauze. After this the whole area is covered with a dressing.

THE CAR ACCIDENT

The Situation

Look for victims: they may be scattered on the road, or out of sight over a hedge.

Inspect the victims quickly for urgent needs (profuse bleeding, asphyxia or burning car). In other circumstances the patient in a car should generally be left where he is. Moving him is best done by the experienced.

Prevent further accident. Attend to the smashed car.

1. Put out fire or smouldering with an extinguisher or by smothering it with a rug, soil or sand. If fire persists get the occupants out quickly lest there be a sudden huge flare. Lie them well away and to windward. Do not smoke.
2. Turn off car lights and switch off the ignition.
3. Apply the brakes, or block the wheels with a bulky object.
4. Set warnings: a red reflector triangle or someone signalling with a torch and a white scarf or newspaper – along the road up to 200 yards either side of the accident, according to terrain and visibility.
5. At night wear something boldly white. Light the scene with headlights of your car placed sideways and off the road. If it has to stay on the road keep the signal lights blinking.

Send for help with a detailed message (see page 154).

The Patient

Beware of the unconscious victim silently in his seat; his neck (perhaps fractured) and his breathing airway are the most vulnerable parts. Both can be protected by supporting neck and jaw with a collar made from a newspaper thickly folded to form a rigid but pliable support about 3 by 12 inches, and inserted into a stocking (kept in your first aid box or sacrificed by a female bystander). Slide the whole under the patient's chin and round his neck; tie the loose ends of the stocking firmly at the rear.

If necessary, while help is being prepared, the slumped patient could be put with his trunk pulled forward and chin resting on his hands, brought together in front of him on steering wheel or dashboard. This also allows fluid present in

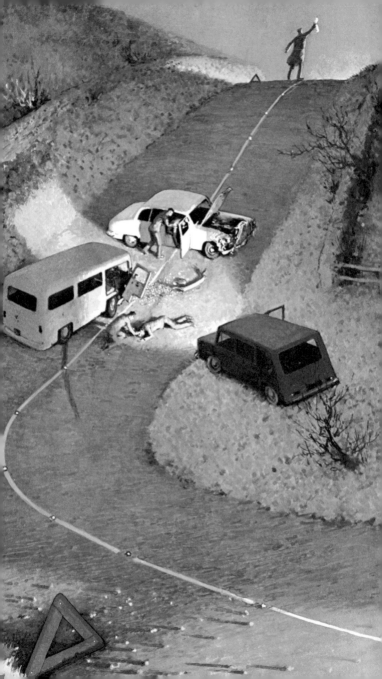

the mouth to drain away. These moves must, of course, be modified if you suspect fractures of upper limbs or chin.

Extracting the patient from a buckled car can be very difficult, especially if the doors are jammed and if the injuries include fractured spine and limbs. Leave it to the experts (police, ambulance, fire brigade, rescue doctors) who carry special equipment, including boards with strapping which let the patient be moved with full protection of an injured spine.

A great deal of immediate first aid such as stopping bleeding or covering wounds can be given to a patient still in the car.

Road smash wounds can be very big and really large dressings should be available. Ideal is Gamgee Tissue, a thick layer of cotton wool sandwiched between two layers of gauze.

The Car First Aid Kit

Keep it in a well closed, but easily opened, clearly labelled, metal or plastic box. Contents should include most or all of the following: triangular bandages (each with safety pin); women's discarded stockings; white gauze; Gamgee Tissue (in large pieces 12 inches by 18 inches); cotton elastic or crepe bandages (3 inches wide); Prepared Sterile Dressings (large size); Adhesive Tape (1 inch wide); a sturdy pair of scissors and a Rescue Blanket (see page 128).

Your car should also carry, as a matter of course, a strong torch, a red reflector triangle and a fire extinguisher.

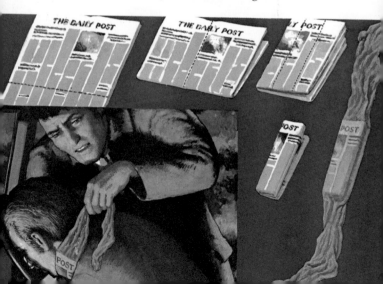

SOME MEDICAL EMERGENCIES

Asthma

This takes many forms, but the usual one is a wheezing struggle to breathe through lung air tubes so narrowed by spasm and internal thickening and discharge that air can hardly pass in and out of the chest.

Potent factors are fear and tension. Reassurance and relaxing are as important as the doctor's drugs. Calm, sympathetic confidence makes a great difference. If the patient is a child give him something to do, even if it is only looking at a book or taking a drink.

Avoid a hot stuffy atmosphere; let in fresh air through open windows unless the weather forbids it. Loosen tight clothing. Breathing is easier with the patient sitting up. For more effective breathing encourage him to make chest movements as deliberately as he can from waist level rather than from higher up. Position him properly, aiming to have his *chest upright*, his *back* straight and his limbs and neck relaxed.

Asthma attack positions. Relax but keep back straight

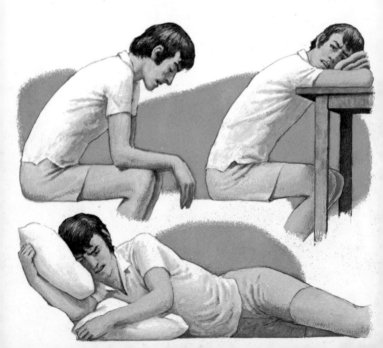

Heart Attack

Under abnormal circumstances the heart's power may suddenly fail; the patient becomes pale or blue with fast breathing which sounds wet or bubbly (not to be confused with the harsh wheeze of asthma).

Another type of attack could arise from serious hindrance to the heart muscles own blood supply. The restricted flow of blood to this muscle causes severe pain in the centre of the chest. Sometimes the pain spreads to shoulders, arms or neck. The patient is likely to be breathless, pale and sweating.

In either case the pulse may be fast and perhaps irregular. Even if the symptoms are milder they must be treated with the same concern. Do not delay in sending for a doctor.

Loosen the patient's clothing and let him choose his easiest position for breathing. Probably this will be sitting up. If he sweats dry his face. However do not fuss him; the man with a heart attack often resents much touching and crowding. Calm reassurance helps a lot.

If the heart stops beating try resuscitation immediately

Asthma attack positions can be achieved out of doors.

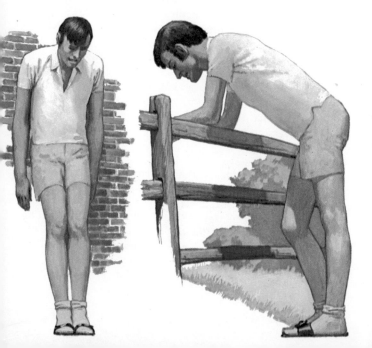

(p. 87). But one cannot overstress the error of giving massage to a heart which is still beating.

Strokes

Strokes are caused by disturbance to a blood vessel of the brain. A clot could cut off the blood supply to the section of brain served by that vessel. Or some brain tissue could be injured by the escape of blood where a vessel has ruptured. Either will impair the functioning of the part of the body governed by that area of the brain. In the same way an accident in a telephone exchange could put out of action those subscribers' telephones which were controlled by the damaged parts of the exchange switchboard.

Therefore the results of a stroke can be extremely variable, ranging from a mild temporary clumsiness of hand, leg or speech to the full loss of power of half the body accompanied by anything from a headache to mental confusion or unconsciousness.

If you suspect a light stroke put the patient at rest in bed and let his doctor know. Keep close watch lest he worsen. More severe cases with bad loss of power, with mental impairment or unconsciousness need medical opinion urgently. Meantime you have the important duty of keeping the patient safe and comfortable and of protecting his breathing by having his head low, by removing false teeth, by wiping away fluid collecting in the mouth and by loosening tight clothes. Keep the unconscious or semi-conscious in the recovery position (page 71).

Remember that the inert and apparently unconscious man may yet hear and judge what you say. Guard your speech.

Epilepsy

Attacks vary a great deal and only an average description can be given. Some begin with a short cry, but generally the episode is quite silent in its four stages.
1. A few epileptics manage to sit or lie down, a special feeling heralding the attack. But the majority suddenly fall unconsciousness, a great danger if they are on stairs, by moving machinery or in traffic.
2. For half to one minute the patient lies motionless with

muscles rigid. He is not breathing and his complexion darkens.

3. Within the next minute jerking appears. Sometimes it starts in one limb before extending to the whole body. These ungoverned movements may make the patient bite his tongue or hit nearby furniture, or cause bowel and bladder to empty. Foam or saliva may appear at the lips.

4. Now the patient relaxes, resumes breathing and lies quietly. He may sleep the attack off for a variable time.

Do not try to control the jerking but let it happen, clearing aside objects which the patient might hit. If he has false teeth try to remove them. Guard against tongue biting by pushing a wedge of folded cloth between the angle of the jaws (use something like the patient's coat lapel if nothing else is available). Wipe away any froth. As soon as the patient has ceased moving put him in the recovery position (see page 71). Also check whether there are outward signs that he hurt himself as he fell.

Hysteria

The hysterical attack makes an excellent comparison and contrast with the epileptic fit. It builds up gradually in an excitable or frustrated person. Consciously or (more likely) unconsciously he is demonstrating his worries. He may not realise or wish to recognise personal anxieties and he turns their effect into a form he can present without psychological discredit as a cry for help and sympathy.

He generally makes a good deal of noise; even if he imitates coma some moans and groans will accompany the act. If he falls he lands safely and comfortably. Movements may range from the pathetically feeble to wild and dramatic waving – quite different from the sustained rapid jerks of epilepsy. He will not soil or wet himself. He will not bite his tongue, for he will be needing it for other purposes. He may complain of peculiar pains or (between hearty breaths) that his respiration has stopped.

Treatment begins with recognising that here is not a real malingerer but a genuinely ill or frightened person and that this is a psychological condition advertising itself in a physical way. It needs an audience.

The first thing to do is to deny the patient that audience by clearing observers out of sight and hearing – especially those solicitous relatives who are showing understandable concern and who will (at first) label you an unfeeling brute.

Examine the patient as briefly as compatible with security. Give reassurance rather than sympathy. Give orders rather than advice. Make statements rather than queries. Be firm rather than pleading. Be a sergeant major rather than a ministering angel. But always reassure.

Do not slap the patient or empty a bucket of cold water on him unless you have a very good solicitor.

Fits in Children

The attack might possibly be an early form of epilepsy but it is much more likely to be the transient effect of fever on the sensitive nervous system of the very young. Rarely fit follows fit, but generally the child comes to rapidly after his one attack. It will have served to alert the parents and get a doctor's attention to the fever.

Follow all the usual measures to keep the airway open and to

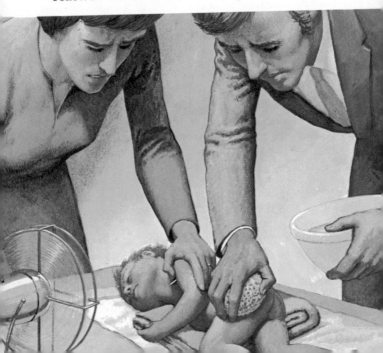

protect breathing. Put the child in the recovery position (page 71). Loosen his clothes, wipe any fluid from his mouth and keep him warm with loose covering. When he has recovered get a doctor's advice.

If the child's temperature is very high remove his clothes, lie him on a towel and sponge gently with cold water. Let this be graded – first the face, then the limbs and last the trunk. Use long smooth strokes and try to let the sponge absorb back water you have pressed out. An electric fan nearby will help. An excessive fall of temperature could cause collapse. Check with a thermometer before and during the sponging. Stop when you have reduced the fever by about one degree Centigrade (two degrees Fahrenheit). Dry the child and cover him with light clothing.

Diabetes

Some foods we eat (especially sweets and starches) are turned into sugar which the body 'burns' as fuel for life. There is always a store of sugar in the body and always a certain amount in the blood (Figure A). The body controls this so that in health the blood's sugar contents always lies between definite upper and lower limits (Figures B and C).

In diabetes this control is lacking and the body has to call upon other substances from its tissues to act as fuel. There are several results. The patient loses weight and becomes very tired. Unused sugar stockpiles in the blood in amounts well above the normal healthy level (Figure D). So high is this concentration that sugar will do what it never does normally; it seeps out of the blood into the kidneys and so into the urine.

Chemical changes resulting from the use of the wrong 'fuel' are slowly poisonous and make the patient more and more lethargic until finally he is very drowsy and may even pass into coma. These changes are *gradual*, spanning many days rather than minutes or hours, giving the patient the chance of consulting his doctor and having the condition diagnosed and treated. The effect of too much sugar forms a medical and not a first aid problem.

Successfully treated, the diabetic's blood sugar returns to normal levels. But to maintain this he is dependent on tablets or injections for he can no longer trust his body to do the

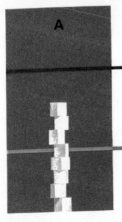

UPPER LIMIT OF NORMAL

LOWER LIMIT OF NORMAL

After a heavy meal the sugar may reach the upper level of normal

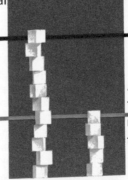

After exertion or fasting the sugar may descend to the lower level of normal

Untreated diabetes with very high sugar level

Treated diabetes in which an abnormally low sugar level occurs

Symptoms develop gradually

Coma may develop rapidly

adjustments automatically. He must adapt himself and his meals to a regular time table so that sugar formed from his foods counterbalance the sugar burning effect of his drugs and vice versa.

If he forgets his drugs or if he eats too much the blood's sugar level will again rise abnormally.

This is quite a minor fault compared to the reverse possibility. If he takes an overdose of his drug or if he exerts himself much more than usual, then far too much 'fuel' will burn up and the sugar level will plunge down below the normal. The same descent could happen if he did not take enough food to balance his usual dose of drugs and exertion (Figure E).

With a level of sugar below the lower value of normal the patient can rapidly become unconscious. Before that he may begin by feeling abnormally hungry or 'hot and cold'. He may be yawning or grimacing. Or he may pass through a phase of being pale, sweating, tremulous, jerky, uncoordinated and stumbling with a thick speech. He could be irrational, perhaps aggressive. In other words he may resemble a drunken man. Once in a coma he may die if not medically treated.

It is in the short precomatose stage, while the patient can still swallow, that the first aider can help. Treatment is simple: give two or three lumps (or teaspoonfuls) of sugar or glucose in water. Repeat this after five minutes if the patient has not improved. He should, in any case, after recovery take a further lot to make sure he does not slip back. If you have no sugar give honey, jam or chocolate. If your patient is shouting and uncooperative a messy but effective dodge is to fling granulated sugar in his mouth each time he opens it.

Most diabetics on treatment have been advised by doctors to carry with them sugar lumps to take if they feel (as some can) a low sugar attack coming on. Not all have the time to do this and finding sugar in the pocket or handbag of an unconscious person may give a clue as to what caused his state. He needs hospital help urgently.

Beware of dismissing the low sugar diabetic casualty as an unpleasant drunk and leaving it at that.

Many diabetics carry in their wallet or pocket a card indicating the diagnosis. It is legitimate to look for this in the unconscious.

THE PATTERN OF FIRST AID

Whoever has studied this far will realise that there is a general shape to the course of treatment. Of course every case is different; in few major first aid incidents can all the points taught be followed completely. Circumstances often may compel one to break the rules deliberately. But rules there are and one should not go wrong if approaching each patient with a programme in mind.

1. If the surroundings themselves are threatening (fire, escaped gas, tottering building) get your patient and your self away as quickly as you can.

2. Otherwise begin by examining and treating the patient where he is. Do not move him until you know what is wrong with him and you feel it is safe to do so.

3. Immediately check:

Has his breathing stopped?	Begin resuscitation
Is he choking?	Clear the airway
Is he bleeding heavily?	Control haemorrhage
Is he unconscious?	Put in the recovery position as soon as you can move him.

4. Prevent the risk of further accidents. Clear the crowd; guard against and control the traffic; remove any dangerous objects such as weapons, lit blow lamps, sharp tools, broken glass. Advise the patient not to move. Protect his property (bag, spectacles, watch) from loss or harm.

5. Reassure the patient. Achieve this by the way you choose your words and the way you say them. Combine consolation with command, and confidence with care. The patient's trust in you and the bystanders' readiness to obey you will depend on the calmness and method of your work.

6. Dress all wounds; immobilise all fractures. Do not forget to check for hidden wounds and unsuspected fractures.

7. Treat to prevent shock whenever necessary.

All the above assumes that you have but one patient. When there are several casualties you must survey very quickly and decide which need your help most urgently. The slightly hurt (with a non bleeding cut, for instance) and those who are severely hurt but not immediately threatened with death (crushed leg or fractured spine) you tell – with reassurance – to remain still until you return to them. You give treatment first to those who could die for lack of rapid action (as in choking, heavy bleeding or chest injury). Decision may be difficult, but your conscience is clear if you try to select priorities instead of taking patients in the order they present.

At this point in your reading it would be well for you to look up again the subjects of internal bleeding (page 32) and head injuries (page 73).

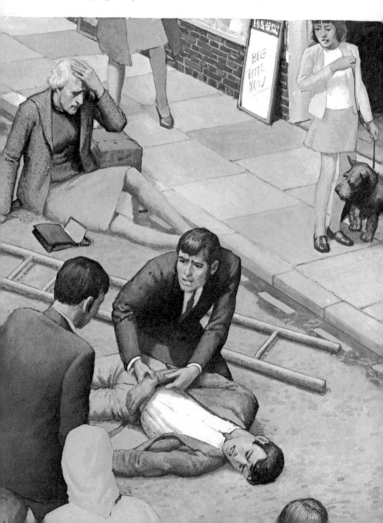

8. Let a suitable bystander be messenger for ambulance or doctor. The message you give him (preferably written) must state very clearly: the site of the accident (house address or field situation for instance) and, if necessary, how to find it (where it is likely to be hard to find post someone by the roadside to signal to and guide ambulance driver or doctor); the number of injured; the nature and also the severity of their injuries; the degree of urgency.

All too often the rescuer sends a panic call without this important information.

9. Gather together any of the patient's property (such as bags, jewellery, dentures, articles of clothing) and hand them to a responsible person or send them with him to hospital.

10. Get the names and addresses of the patients sent to hospital and make sure that their relatives receive a tactful message. If the police come on the scene they will undertake this.

11. After you have completed the treatment and while you await others who will take charge, stay near the patient and watch him lest he worsen.

12. Whenever an incident may possibly have later legal or official consequences keep careful notes about the injury, the patient's condition and your actions. Date and time them. Memory is fallible and details written like this *at the time or immediately after* can be immensely valuable if any queries arise or if you have to give evidence in court, perhaps months afterwards.

We now have learnt that First Aid consists not just of attending to a patient but, more broadly, of coping with a situation.

First Aid Kit for the Home

Everything should be held in a metal or plastic box which closes properly but is easy to open. Label it properly and keep it in a place known to all the household but well out of the reach of children. Anything you use from it you should replace as soon as possible.

The contents may be made up from:

white gauze, cotton wool, paper tissues (in small unopened packs); *plain bandages*, 2 and 3 inches; *cotton crepe bandage* (slightly elastic and can shape round and support a limb, 3 inches); *heavy cotton elastic bandage* (thicker and firmer for good pressure, 3 inches); *perforated film absorbent* ('P.F.A.') *dressings* (4 or 2 inches square, sterile and wrapped individually in protective envelopes – can be removed and put on without being touched by hand. The *shiny* surface goes on the wound); *adherent dressing strips* (2 or 3 inches width, can be cut to size for covering simple wounds); *tubular gauze bandage* (illustrated) (comes with an applicator which allows neat bandaging over dressings of toes and fingers. Size 01 (small) and 12 (big) and applicator size 1 will do for both); *prepared sterile dressing* (illustrated) (a thick dressing pad with bandage attached. Put the pad on the wound, wind round the short bandage strip from one end, then cover the whole by winding the long bandage from the other end in the opposite direction. The large size with its pad of 6 inches square is recommended); *triangular bandages* (see page 59); *adhesive strapping* 1 inch wide; *safety pins*; *tweezers* with fine points; *scissors* (kept sharp and for first aid only); *thermometer* (see page 126); Cetrimide solution 1%, Cetrimide cream $\frac{1}{2}$% (see page 48); *antihistamine cream* (see page 136); *soluble aspirin or paracetamol tablets* for use against pain.

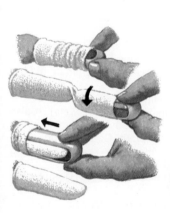
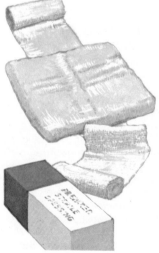

ACKNOWLEDGEMENTS

The author is very grateful to colleagues who kindly let him benefit from their advice and specialist experience: Dr. K. C. Easton; Dr. E. F. Edson; Miss Diana Gaskell M.C.S.P.; Surgeon Lieutenant-Commander F. St. C. Golden, R.N.; Mr. P. S. London, F.R.C.S.; Dr. O. J. Ófeigsson of Reykjavik; Mr. Christopher Parish, F.R.C.S.

The illustration on page 41 is based on a photograph from Dr. Ófeigsson published in the British Journal of Plastic Surgery; that on page 81 was developed from a teaching of Mr. London; the positions shown on pages 144, 145 were inspired by the work of Physiotherapy Department of the Brompton Hospital, London.

FIRST AID COURSES

The three major organisations which run such courses are:
The St. John Ambulance Association, 1 Grosvenor Crescent, London S.W.1.
The St. Andrew's Ambulance Association, Milton Street, Glasgow C.4.
The British Red Cross Society, 9 Grosvenor Crescent, London S.W.1.
An enquiry to these Headquarters (or a look in the telephone book) will obtain the address of the local branch.

BOOKS TO STUDY

First Aid Manual, 3rd edition 1972. The official text book jointly issued by the three organisations listed above. It is a 'must' for anyone who aims to pass their examination (and everyone should!)
First Aid Junior Manual, 11th edition 1972 is issued by the British Red Cross Society for junior students (cadets). It also forms a useful brief-style summary for adults.
New Advanced First Aid by A. Ward Gardner and P. J. Roylance, Butterworths, 1969, offers the keenly enquiring first aider a clear and deep insight into techniques.
Sports Injuries by D. S. Mukle, Onet Press, 1971. Useful for the man attending a team.
Road Accidents Medical Aid by Hanns Pacy, Livingstone, 1971, is almost a necessity today.
Principles of First Aid for the Injured by H. Proctor and P. S. London, 2nd edition, Butterworths, 1968, and *Emergency*

Care 7th edition, edited by W. H. Cole and C. B. Prestow, Butterworths, 1972 are respectively from Britain and America. They give advanced technical views of first aid and of the immediate surgical or medical second aid beyond it.

INDEX

Page numbers set in **bold** type refer to illustrations

Abdominal wounds, 48–9, **49**
Air passages, clearance of, 68–9, 79, **68, 69**
Agricultural poisons, 122–3
Ankle, **66**
  dislocated, **67**
  fractured, **67**
  sprained, 11, **66**
Antiseptics, 48
Arm,
  bleeding from, 34–7, **35, 36**
  fracture of, 57, 59, **56, 57**
Artificial respiration, 84, 86, 87, 88–99, 100, 101, 116
  Holger Nielsen method of, 88, 96–7, **97**
  mouth-to-mouth method of, 88, 89–95, **88, 90, 91, 92, 93**
  mouth-to-nose method of, 92–3
  Silvester method of, 88, 98–9, **88, 98, 99**
Asthma attacks, 144, **144, 145**

Bandaging, 26, 46, 49, 50, 135, **26, 135**
Bites, snake, 137–8
Bleeding, 6–9, 23–37, 72
  (see also individual sources of bleeding)
  internal, 32–3
  shock and, 6–9
  stopping, 24–6, 95, **24**
Blisters, 9, 140, **39, 140**
Blood,
  clotting, 24
  functions of, 37
  volume, 6–7, 23, **6**
Brain compression, 75–9, **75, 76**
Breathing, 22, 72, 82–105, **106**
  cessation of, 82–4

  obstruction of, 68, 72, 84–5, **68, 69, 84**
  first aid for, 85, **86**
Bruising, 10–11, 81, **10, 81**
  and shock, 10–11
Bullet wounds, 46
Burns 38–43, **39, 40, 41, 42**
  chemical, 42–3
  damage caused by, 39–40
  electrical, 43, 114
  first aid to, 40–2
  friction, 43
  of clothes, 38–9
  shock and, 9

Car accidents, 107, 141–3, **142, 143**
Carbon dioxide, 82, 94, 95
Carbon monoxide
  poisoning, 87–8, 100, 116–7
Cetrimide 45, 48
Chemical burns, 42–3
Chest, injuries to, 106–10, **107, 108, 109**
Childbirth, 130–4, **131, 133, 134**
  preparations for, **131**
Choking, 84, 85, 87
Cold reactions, 127–9
Collar bone, fracture of, 56
Concussion, 74, 77–9
Coughing, 84
Cramped muscles, 136
Crush injury 50
Crushed chest 107
Cuts, 10, 44, **44**

Diabetes, 149–51
Dislocation, 66–7, **67**
Dressings, 25, 28, 41, 44–6, 154–5, **25, 26, 155**
Drinks,
  after burns, 42
  after poisoning, 121
  after injury, 21, 50
  warm, after exposure,

127, 128
Drowning, 87, 95

Ear,
    bleeding from, 27–8, **27**
    objects in, 138
Electrical burns, 43, **43**
Electric shocks, 88, 111–4
    first aid for, 112–4 **113**
Emotional shock, 5
Epilepsy, 146–7
Evidence in court 154
Exposure, 127–8
Eyes,
    effect of brain
        compression on, 77
    objects in, 139–40, **139**
    wounds of, 48

First aid,
    definition of, 4
    general rules of, 152–4
    kits, 143, 154–5
    organisations, 4–5, 156, **5**
    teaching of, 5
Fits, in children, 148–9, **148**
Foot, fracture of, 61, **61**
Fractures, 11, 51–65 (see
        also individual bones)
    blood loss from, 11, **13**
    closed, 52, **52**
    complicated, 54, **52, 53**
    direct, 51–2, **51**
    first aid for, 54–65, **56,
        57, 58, 59, 60, 61**
    immobilisation of, 54–6,
        55
    indirect, 52, **51**
    muscular, 52
    open, 52, 54, **52**
    shock and, 11
    sites of, **53**
    spontaneous, 52
Friction burns, 43
Frostbite, 127

Gas poisoning, 116
Grazes, 44, **44**

Hand,
    bleeding from, 34–7, **36**
    fracture of, 57
Hanging, 85
Head injuries, 73–81
    first aid for, 79–81
Heart,
    attacks, 88, 145–6
    massage, 87, 89, 100–5,
        102, 103, 104, 105

Heat,
    exhaustion, 124–5, **124**
    stroke, 125–6, **125**
Hip, fracture of, 62, **62**
Holger Nielsen method (see
        artificial respiration)
Hypothermia, 128–9
Hysteria, 147

Insect stings, 136
Internal,
    bleeding, 32–3
    injuries, 81

Jaw, fracture of, 61

Lacerations, 10, 44, **44**
Legs, fracture of, 60–1, **60**
Lightning shocks, 88, 114,
    115
Lungs, 82, **83**
    bleeding from, 30, 106,
        107
injuries to, 106–10

Miscarriage, 134
Mouth,
    scalding of, 43
    -to-mouth method (see
        artificial respiration)
    -to-nose method (see
        artificial respiration)
Muscles, 51, **50**
    cramped, 136
    strained, 135–6, **135**

Nerve shock, 5
Nose,
    bleeding from, 28
    objects in, 138

Oxygen 82, 94

Pelvis, fracture of, 62, **62**
Poisoning, 87–8,
    116–23
    agricultural, 122–3
    carbon monoxide, 116, 118
    first aid for, 116–22, **117**
    prevention of, **118, 120,
        123**
Pressure points, 34–7, **35**
Primary shock, 5
Pulse rate, 22–3
    effect of brain
        compression on, 77

taking the, 22–3, 100–1,
23, 100

Recovery position 69–71,
71
Red Cross, badge of, **5**
Rescue Blanket, 128
Resuscitation, 87–105, 112
*(see also artificial
respiration and heart
massage)*
Ribs, fracture of, 57

St. Andrews, badge of, **5**
St. John, badge of, **5**
Scalds, 42, 43
Shock, 5–22
  bleeding and, 6–9
  bruising and, 10–11
  burns and, 10–11
  causes of, 6–11
  classification of, 5–6
  development of, **8**
  fractures and, 11
  prevention of, 13–22,
  14
  symptoms of, 13
  wounds and, 10–11
Shrapnel wounds, 46
Silvester method *(see
artificial respiration)*
Skin, burning of, 39, **39, 41**
Skull, 73, **73**
  fracture of, 27, 28, 74–5,
  74
Slings, 59, **58, 59**
Snakes,
  bites of, 137–8
Spine, fracture of, 62–5, **64,
65**
Sprains, 66–7
Stings, 136
Stomach, bleeding from,
  30–1, **31, 32**

Stove-in chest, 107
Strained muscles, 135–6,
  135
Strangling, 84, 87
Strokes, 146
Suffocation, 84, 87
Swelling, caused by
  bleeding, 10, 11

Temperature,
  changes, 124–9
  reduction of, 126
Tetanus, 48
Thermometer,
  hypothermia, 129, **129**
  values, **126**
Throat, scalding of, 43
Tongue, bleeding from, 29
Tooth socket, bleeding
  from, 29

Unconsciousness, 68–81,
  85, 128
  first aid for, 69–72, **68,
  69, 70**

Varicose veins, bleeding
  from, 33
Vomit, 31

Wounds, 10–11, 44–9, 81
  *(see also specific areas
  and types)*
  antiseptics and, 48
  cleaning of, 45, 46, **45**
  embedded objects in, 46,
  47
  first aid to, 44–6
  shock and, 10–11
  tetanus and, 48
Wrist,
  bleeding from, 34–7
  fracture of, 57

SOME OTHER TITLES IN THIS SERIES

- Arts
- Domestic Animals and Pets
- Domestic Science
- Gardening
- General Information
- History and Mythology
- Natural History
- Popular Science

Arts
Antique Furniture/Architecture/Clocks and Watches/Glass for Collectors/Jewellery/Musical Instruments/Porcelain/Pottery/Victoriana

Domestic Animals and Pets
Budgerigars/Cats/Dog Care/Dogs/Horses and Ponies/Pet Birds/Pets for Children/Tropical Freshwater Aquaria/Tropical Marine Aquaria

Domestic Science
Flower Arranging

Gardening
Chrysanthemums/Garden Flowers/Garden Shrubs/House Plants/Plants for Small Gardens/Roses

General Information
Aircraft/Arms and Armour/Coins and Medals/Flags/Fortune Telling/Freshwater Fishing/Guns/Military Uniforms/Motor Boats and Boating/National Costumes of the World/Orders and Decorations/Rockets and Missiles/Sailing/Sailing Ships and Sailing Craft/Sea Fishing/Trains/Veteran and Vintage Cars/Warships

History and Mythology
Age of Shakespeare/Archaeology/Discovery of: Africa/The American West/Australia/Japan/North America/South America/Great Land Battles/Great Naval Battles/Myths and Legends of: Africa/Ancient Egypt/Ancient Greece/Ancient Rome/India/The South Seas/Witchcraft and Black Magic

Natural History
The Animal Kingdom/Animals of Australia and New Zealand/Animals of Southern Asia/Bird Behaviour/Birds of Prey/Butterflies/Evolution of Life/Fishes of the world/Fossil Man/A Guide to the Seashore/Life in the Sea/Mammals of the world/Monkeys and Apes/Natural History Collecting/The Plant Kingdom/Prehistoric Animals/Seabirds/Seashells/Snakes of the world/Trees of the world/Tropical Birds/Wild Cats

Popular Science
Astronomy/Atomic Energy/Chemistry/Computers at Work/The Earth/Electricity/Electronics/Exploring the Planets/Heredity The Human Body/Mathematics/Microscopes and Microscopic Life/Physics/Undersea Exploration/The Weather Guide